MATT DELITO is a 30-something constable in the Metropolitan Police. He switched careers relatively late – exchanging spreadsheets, a Ford Focus rep car and a pretty decent salary for paperwork, a Ford Focus (but this time one with blue lights on the roof), and a far less decent salary.

And yet, he's much happier for it.

MATT DELITO

Confessions of a Police Constable

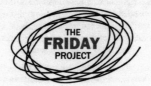

The Friday Project
An imprint of HarperCollins*Publishers*
77–85 Fulham Palace Road
Hammersmith
London W6 8JB

www.harpercollins.co.uk

This edition published by The Friday Project in 2013

ISBN: 978-0-00-749745-4

Set in Minion by Palimpsest Book Production Limited,
Falkirk, Stirlingshire

Printed and bound in Great Britain by
Clays Ltd, St Ives plc

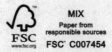

MIX
Paper from
responsible sources
FSC
www.fsc.org
FSC® C007454

The stories in this book describe my experiences working as a police constable in London. To protect confidentiality, not everything I write can be one hundred per cent *the truth, the whole truth, and nothing but the truth* – some parts have been fictionalised, and names and locations have been changed. I'm unable to share some of my favourite stories because they are part of investigations in progress. Others I must amend slightly because I don't want to put my colleagues at risk by revealing operationally sensitive information. Most importantly, I really like my job, and I would rather not get dismissed.

Who am I?

Hi, my name is Matt Delito.

I am a police officer in London's Metropolitan Police Force. *Service*. I mean Service. In the immortal words of Nicholas Angel in *Hot Fuzz* – which, incidentally, should certainly be introduced as mandatory viewing for new recruits to the Metropolitan Police – 'We're not calling it a "police force" any more; that's too aggressive.'

You don't have to call us the Metropolitan Police Service, or even the MPS – 'The Met' will do. Of course, I'm aware that people have an awful lot of other names for us, but many of them aren't fit to print in a fine publication such as this.

When I'm on duty, I am usually on 'team'. This is short for 'response team'. We're the guys who come rushing to your assistance when someone breaks into your house and you dial 999. The borough I work in is one of the busiest in London, and I'm part of one of the best teams around. If we are on duty, and you live, work or play in my part of town, you're in good hands . . .

Okay, I haven't been entirely upfront: my name isn't, in fact, Matt Delito, although it does have a pretty good ring to it. And my collar number is not PC592MD, and I am not based at

Southwark (which is what an 'MD' shoulder number would usually indicate).

If it turns out there's a PC592MD: I'm sorry, buddy, the number was picked at random.

Matt Delito

Pleased to meet you . . .

I was slumped back against a tree stump at the edge of the park, watching the two youths run off into the distance. I was only dimly aware of the electronic device I was holding in my hand.

'Hello? Hello!?'

The little machine was making sounds, but they barely registered in my consciousness. Somehow, I made out the noise of my watch beeping twice, signifying that it was 3 a.m.

'This,' I thought to myself, 'has been a particularly rotten day.'

But I'm getting ahead of myself – introductions first.

I'm Matt.

I'm a police officer, but I haven't always been. I've had quite a few different jobs in my time, including working in a petrol station (I would tell you that it was a barrel of laughs if it wasn't such an easy-to-detect lie). I also worked as a runner for the BBC one particularly memorable summer. That was exciting; I got to meet all sorts of interesting people. Jeremy Clarkson, for example. He told me to fuck off once, which was probably the highlight of my pre-police career. I suppose that goes some way towards explaining why I prefer to talk about my career on the force than about life before I zipped up my Kevlar Metvest for the first time.

I'd like to invite you, for a minute, to think about what your average day consists of. No, go on, I'll just sit back and have a few sips of my coffee whilst you ponder. Unless you're my OP/IRV (this is the operator – aka the person who isn't the driver – on an Incident Response Vehicle), your days will probably be slightly different from mine.

But what *do* I do all day? When I got tired of explaining this to my enquiring friends (and listening to their complaints about police officers: 'I don't like you lot – you gave my sister a ticket for speaking on her mobile when she was driving'), I decided it was time I started writing some of it down. That was well over a year ago now, and the result is the stack of dead trees, or the weightless, electron-powered virtual version thereof you are holding in your hands.

But I digress.

Where was I? Oh, yes, slumped against a tree.

I had just come off duty after a particularly long and dreary shift. It was late on a hot but rapidly cooling July evening and I was cycling home. Yes, 'cycling'. I would not normally cycle so late but my motorbike had been involved in an unfortunate run-in with a bin lorry whilst it was parked outside the police station. I can't really be sure that it was an accident rather than a particularly potent anti-police lash-out, but either way, the result was that my poor motorbike was stuck at the Yamaha dealership, and I was downgraded from triple-digit horsepower to zero-point-not-a-lot of horsepower, sweating and swearing in equal measure as I wrestled my pushbike along the godforsaken bicycle paths.

I was cycling through the park, through the dark, through the night, when out of the corner of my eye, I spotted some movement. At nearly 3 a.m., in a less-than-glamorous slice of town, movement generally signifies bad news, so I slowed down to take a closer look.

Slowing down, as it turned out, might very well have been a good idea; it may have saved my life, in fact. The next thing I knew, I was thrown from my bicycle. It transpired that the movement I'd noticed was a teenager ducking behind a tree, after he and a friend had spanned a length of steel wire across the cycle path, at roughly neck level.

This is an old trick: get the cyclist off the bike and then nick their bike and possessions whilst they are dazed and confused. Or, in some particularly unfortunate cases, dead.

As I lay flat on my back, the two youths came out of the darkness. One of them grabbed my bike, jumped on, and pedalled like a youth possessed into the night. The other quickly dug through my pockets, before running after his friend with my gym bag in his hand.

'Hello? Is there anybody there? Can I help you? What is your emergency?'

I looked down at my hand.

My old, crappy Nokia was gripped between my fingers – clearly the thieves had not wanted it. The screen was lit up. It read 999. I realised that I must have dialled the emergency number, despite my barely sentient state.

'Hello, this is Matt Delito, I'm a police constable, Mike Delta five-nine-two.' I gave the operator my shoulder number completely automatically; I'm not actually sure whether they cared in the slightest.

'I've just been attacked with a garrotte wire in the park by two youths. Both are IC1[1], around sixteen years of age, slim builds, just over five foot tall, both wearing black tracksuits. One had white trainers; the other was wearing a baseball cap. A red one, I think. Also, I need LAS. I think I may have broken my wrist.' LAS are my brothers in arms: the London Ambulance Service.

---

[1] IC stands for Identity Code. They are used to describe the apparent ethnic background of Victims, Informants, Witnesses and Suspects (collectively known as VIWS). IC1 means 'white'.

Within moments of giving my details to the 999 operator, I heard the sirens of a passing police car flick on, and before long saw the silhouettes of my trusty colleagues Pete and Kim running towards me. A second car showed up minutes later with two more of my colleagues, and more importantly one of my assailants – the one with the red baseball cap.

I was still on the ground, heart pounding, with a god-awful pain in my wrist. I looked up at the young man being paraded towards me.

'You've made a few pretty big mistakes today, young man,' I said, as he half-heartedly struggled against his handcuffs.

'You're lucky I am tall,' I continued. 'If I'd been six inches shorter, that cable could have taken my windpipe off, and you would have found yourself staring at a prison wall for the foreseeable future.'

I didn't have the heart to tell him that his other mistake was not stealing my little Nokia. It's hardly the fanciest piece of equipment, but being able to dial 999 immediately was probably the only reason the boy was caught. If I had waited for even a couple of minutes, I have no doubt they would have got away with it.

The boy was bundled into a caged van a few minutes later. I sighed: I had already done a 14-hour shift, but I knew I'd be spending the next ten hours having my wrist set at the hospital, being lectured about concussions, giving witness statements back at the police station, and shaking my head at the idiocy of it all.

The arm hurt, and my chest ached from where the wire had cut into it. I'll be honest with you, though: most of all, I was pissed off that I wouldn't get a good night's sleep.

God knows I needed one.

Can't we all just be friends?

'I want him out of here,' the woman screeched, as she reached over my shoulder, the fingers of her hand curled into a claw, and her impressively long nails slashing, musketeer-style, through the air in the direction of her partner.

'Shut it, you fucking whore,' he barked back, and made a break for her, his hands balled into fleshy, white-knuckled fists.

I deduced from the trickle of blood coming from the man's face that she'd managed to land at least a few scratches before we'd made it into the flat. Her face told a tale as well: her eye was practically swelling up as we stood there.

Seven minutes earlier, we'd received a call over the radio: 'Domestic in progress, graded I, India.'

Our calls are graded in three levels of urgency: E-grade (or Echo) is, basically, whenever you can find the time to rock up. Court warnings, routine appointments and simple follow-ups tend to be graded E. The next step up is an S-grade (or Sierra), where we are meant to make it to the caller within the hour. Dealing with shoplifters, looking for suspicious persons, anything not super-urgent gets a Sierra grade.

Finally we have the most urgent calls, graded I, India. I-graded calls have to be responded to within 12 minutes, so that's when my advanced driving gets put to the test. The flashing lights go on, the sirens are dusted off and put to good use, and my engine and brakes get a good workout.

This time, the address that showed up on the MDT[2] as relayed by the CAD[3] operator made my heart sink. I knew the house well. It belonged to one of those couples that 'love each other' so much that they seem to celebrate their passion largely through beating seven bells out of each other after consuming a drink or 18 between them.

We would attend this address at least a couple of times per month. The training school at Hendon[4] loves to remind us that 'domestic violence intervention is murder prevention', but I've got to admit to having thought more than once that perhaps we should just leave this particular couple to it. For as long as I have been a copper in this borough, they seem to have been completely hell-bent on putting new dents into each other, and it's a pitiful mess every time.

'Take him away! I don't want him here,' she squealed, as I walked in through the front door.

I was the second car on scene, which is just as well, because I'm single-crewed. The car that beat me there was triple-crewed – unusual, given that, in these times of relentless belt-tightening, we're usually one-up in a car, not three. I was glad to see that my colleague Tim was there; he knows the couple well. In addition to Tim, there was Charlie, a relatively new probationer, fresh out of Hendon, and Syd, a special constable.

Specials are volunteers. Many people seem to confuse them with PCSO[5] staff, but there are crucial differences between them,

---

[2] Mobile Data Terminal

[3] Computer Aided Dispatch

[4] Hendon Police College, a huge training complex that serves as the main campus for the Metropolitan Police.

[5] Police Community Support Officer

the main one being that special constables don't get paid. Also, not many people realise this, but special constables have the same powers as myself: they have been sworn in, are warranted by the Queen to do arrests, talk sternly to inebriated teenagers, wag their fingers at people failing to wear seat belts, heroically rescue kittens out of trees, and so on and so forth.

I sneak a look at this particularly solidly built special's Metvest. I think I've seen him before, but I can't remember his name; his nametag reads Smith, which is profoundly unhelpful.

He was doing his best to keep the man from getting to his lady-love. Meanwhile, Tim was trying to reason with the woman, in the hope she would come down from being a squeaky, hyper-ventilating ball of fury.

'Oi!' I called out. 'Can we all just shut up for ten seconds? I can't hear myself think in this racket.'

Weirdly (and unusually), they listened to me. The flat fell quiet for a couple of seconds, except for the man's heavy breathing, leaving all six of us staring back and forth at each other for a few seconds.

'Right,' I said, taking control of the situation in the brief moment of silence. 'You—,' I pointed at the man, 'let's go to the living room and have a chat.'

Tim started leading the woman out of the kitchen and into the bedroom. Good thinking. Kitchens are the most dangerous rooms in a house when there's a chance a fight will break out. Heavy pans, plenty of knives, boiling water – it rarely ends well.

I waved the special over to me, and after we'd had a brief chat with the king of this particularly squalid castle, we explained to him that he needed to be arrested so we would be able to interview him properly. I decided to let the special get the body (which is police slang for 'making the arrest'), mostly for my own amuse-ment, but he promptly ruined my entertainment by knowing what to do, and the arrest went smoothly.

Or at least, it looked to be going smoothly . . . until the man suddenly changed his mind. Immediately after the special applied one handcuff to him, he decided he didn't want to get arrested after all. At first, he started struggling half-heartedly, but then he found some strength and with it a burst of uninhibited inspiration for mayhem. He booted the special in the shins, and managed to swipe my legs from under me. I hit the floor with a rib-crunching crash, hitting the back of my head against the side of a table. Pain shot through me briefly, before fading away again.

'For Christ's sake,' I shouted. In response, the probationer – PC McOwen – came running to help us out. And so developed an all-out fight between the three of us and the man. The TV was kicked – I have no idea by whom – and crashed into the wall. Chairs were knocked over, a series of pictures that were balanced on a shelf went flying across the living room, covering the floor in shards of glass, and the table I had already landed on once ended up in several pieces on the floor.

Amid the chaos I heard McOwen scream, 'SPRAY, SPRAY.'

He had taken his CS spray out of its holder, and was applying a generous dose of noxious liquid (which is not entirely dissimilar to pepper spray) to the man's face.

The man calmed down rapidly, which is great news, obviously, but in the process, I caught some of the CS splash-back, and my eyes filled with tears and a burning sensation I haven't felt since *The Stag Do That Must Not Be Mentioned*.

I react terribly to CS. Generally, I'd prefer we didn't use the stuff in any circumstances. In the probationer's defence, I suppose it was rather effective in this case; chances are we would have continued our living-room-trashing wrestling session for at least a couple of minutes more.

We finally managed to get the man in both cuffs, lying on the floor with the special constable sitting on his legs, the man reeling off a vituperation of obscenities about our mothers, and the probationer holding the handcuffs.

Having reached this position of relative control, we allowed ourselves to relax. It was all over, right?

Right?

Rarely do we have such luck; charging out of the bedroom came the man's girlfriend, holding a rather large box set of the TV series *Friends*.

Yes, really.

'Leave him alone, he hasn't done anything to you,' she shouted, before lifting the box set above her head, and bringing it down on the special.

Tim came running into the living room after her – I am still not sure how she managed to give him the slip – and tried to grab her. She struggled violently, elbowing him in the face and sending him to the floor. Yowling like a doom-wraith she hit the special with the box set again, this time with enough force that it disintegrated. A flurry of CDs, booklets and bits of torn box flew everywhere.

Between the four of us, we restrained her as well, and started taking the man out of the flat, where a caged police van had just arrived with further reinforcements and a way of transporting the fine specimen of gentlemanhood to a night in the cells.

As we hauled the man off, the woman was roaring from within Tim and McOwen's grasp.

'LOVE YOU,' she called to her partner, before directing her anger at us. 'You are hurting him, I love him, leave him alone!' she half-sobbed, half-shouted, conveniently forgetting her insistence that we take him away not ten minutes earlier.

We arranged another van to take her away as well, and they both spent the rest of the night in separate cells, shouting across the hallway between the cells, declaring their mutual undying love approximately 68 times, much to the chagrin of the sleep-deprived custody sergeant.

The next day, lover-boy woke up to yet another ABH (Actual Bodily Harm) charge for beating up his girlfriend for the hundredth time. Meanwhile she was awarded with an assault charge for her valiant rescue attempt.

Before long they were back in the flat, continuing on their previous path of loving each other to death.

The A-hole who dropped the N-bomb

'Hey, Delito,' the sarge said to me that morning, in the daily briefing. 'Thompson is off ill today, can you take care of the Sierra Delta gang?'

Sierra Delta – or SD – is Street Duties. It is a programme where new police officers are put through their paces, dealing with cases from beginning to end. They might do an arrest for a shoplifting, for example, and go through the whole process, from alpha to omega. Arrest, booking into custody, interview on tape, investigation, and so on and so forth: the whole process right through to court. It means that each case you deal with takes a lot of time, but you also get a full understanding of how the processes work. It's incredibly interesting, and I recall my street-duty sessions fondly – the PC who was my mentor/instructor is still one of my best friends to this day.

'Delito. You listening?' Daydreaming already? Oh dear, today really was going to be a long day.

'Sure thing, sarge, I'll do my best,' I replied.

At the end of the briefing, I headed over to the classroom to meet Sasha and Pete, the street duties probationers. They were coming up to the end of their street duties, and they generally had their ducks in a row.

Pete is one of those people who seem to be fuelled purely by air and love for The Job. He also has a look that – when combined with the uniform – makes women swoon when they see him. In some officers – the ones able to pretend they don't notice, or don't know – that can be a fantastic trait, because it makes certain quick quests for information all that much quicker. Pete knows what he's doing, and he's a solid police officer. If the women think 'He can fuck me', the men think 'He can fuck me up'. In short, Pete spends every minute he doesn't spend in uniform in a gym. I've run into him at the gym a couple of times, and he doesn't mess around; he may very well be the fittest officer on the entire borough. He's not particularly tall – about five foot seven – but he's built like a row of brick-and-mortar outhouses, and inspires confidence through and through.

Sasha is not entirely unlike Pete in many ways: she's witty, knows her laws and white notes[6] inside out, and she's no slouch either – she regularly runs half marathons and is apparently trying for her taekwondo black belt. She's about as tall as Pete. Her slender build, short hair and fragile-looking glasses make her positively androgynous-looking – especially when she's fully kitted out in her Metvest. She famously disposed of the rumours of her being a lesbian by sleeping with Pete just for long enough that everybody knew about it, before dumping him and returning to single life. The 'everybody knew about it' part was secured when she, early one Tuesday morning, transmitted over the radio, on the open channel, 'Mike Delta two-two-three, do you have any johnnies?'

She got into some trouble with the brass about that one, but she gained major points with the rest of the team, and she's now well known as someone who doesn't mince her words – quite refreshing, really.

Once we've all said our hellos, we sit down briefly and talk

---

[6] The training paperwork you get when you learn everything you need to know to be a police officer.

about some questions they have, before breaking out the boot polish, giving our shoes a quick shine, and hitting the streets. Street duties involve a lot of foot patrolling, so you get a proper workout in the process, but seeing as I spend most of my time either driving around in a car or doing quick sprints after naughty little toe-rags, I usually find a walking session to be no bad thing.

It was a pretty slow morning. The radio was so dead that people occasionally ran a radio check, just to make sure their radios hadn't stopped working. So, without anything better to do, we decided to head out on 'reassurance patrol'.

Reassurance patrolling is usually done in areas where something bad has happened recently. Not long ago, we'd had a series of stabbings in one particular part of the borough, so we decided we'd take a stroll down the streets that had been worst affected, stop to have a chat with some of the shop owners, and just see how things were looking, on the whole.

By the time the morning had crawled to an end, we'd handed out five traffic tickets (all for mobile phone use), taken weed off some young troublemakers and issued them with a formal warning, and spent a bit of time running after a shoplifter who was unlucky enough to come across our path, before continuing his unlucky streak by running straight into a blind alley, where Sasha quickly got her arrest in. We dealt with it swiftly – both Pete and Sasha had made dozens of arrests by this point – and once we were done, we decided to pop into KFC for some lunch.

This particular branch of the Kentucky Fried Chicken (or Unlucky Fried Kitten, as we tend to call it round these parts) is weirdly L-shaped, and we took our seats in the short leg of the 'L' to chomp down our meals.

As we were idly chatting, we heard some commotion by the counter. When we'd come in, we had spotted a security guard, so I figured he'd take care of things. But no such luck: things escalated rapidly.

'I gave you 40 pounds, you fat bitch.' A voice broke through to our table of three, ending our genteel luncheon abruptly. Sasha and Pete looked at each other, then at me.

'Hey, you are the cops,' I said, grinning, as I took the last bite of my Zinger Tower meal. With a full mouth, I continued, 'Go deal with it.'

The dashing duo rounded the corner, with me following a few steps behind.

Leaning forward with one hand on the counter was a very large man in a bright patterned shirt. When I say large, I mean very, very large indeed. Positively obese, in fact – larger than any man I had ever seen before in my life. For every movement he made with his arm, another part of his body seemed to be moving, as if it were echoing it – or perhaps protesting under its own weight.

Behind him was a shorter but no less formidable woman, who turned out to be his wife. The couple were on their honeymoon from Texas and had decided to come to London 'because we love musicals', they told me at some point later in the proceedings.

I recognised the man's accent as American, but I wasn't really sure who he had shouted at. In addition to the couple, the security guard was standing very close to them, making sounds designed – but failing – to calm them down.

'What's going on here?' Sasha interrupted.

'Ah, thank fuck for that,' the man exclaimed. 'This fat bitch stole my money,' he repeated. I half expected him to point to his wife, but he nodded to the serving counter. I looked. At first glance, the counter was empty, but then I spotted a girl – not older than 20 – cowering behind one of the fryers.

'Excuse me, could you come out,' Pete said, waving to the girl for her to come closer, and smiling that broad, winning smile of his. 'We just want to find out what's been going on here.'

Pete was in front of me, so I have no idea what he was doing, but based on how the girl reacted, I can't help but think that he must at least have winked at her. For the briefest of moments, I entertained myself with the idea that he might conceivably have blown her a kiss.

The girl – her nametag revealed her name to be Cecilie – was five feet tall at the most. She could probably do with going jogging every now and again, perhaps, but calling her 'fat' hardly seemed fair, especially considering the girth of both the man and his wife. As soon as Cecilie stepped out, the man went off on one again.

'I paid you forty pounds! You gave me change for thirty! Where is my change, you dim-witted bitch?' the man hissed.

'Hey,' said the security guard, wearily, 'There's no need for that kind of language. We have CCTV covering all the cash registers, and can easily check whether you got short-changed. If that's the case, we'll of course make sure you get the right change.'

The way the security guard had taken control of the situation was admirable, a perfect example of conflict resolution: admit there may have been a mistake, offer to look into it, and propose a resolution. Surely, nobody could have a problem with that?

Very, very slowly, with all the eager acceleration of an iceberg, the man turned around, and took a couple of tiny, shuffling steps towards the security guard. The only reason they weren't nose-to-nose was that the guest's remarkably sized stomach prevented him from getting any closer.

'Fuck you, you fucking nigger,' the customer sneered, followed by what seemed an eternity of silence. The security guard just stared at him. I expected him to be angry, but instead he was completely shocked. Even working as a security guard in a fast-food restaurant in a relatively gritty part of town, he didn't experience 'the N word' all that often.

'Right, that's it,' Sasha said. 'I'm arresting you for offences under sections 4a and 18 of the public order act. You do not have to say anything, but it may harm your defence if, when questioned, you fail to mention something you later rely on in court. Anything you do say may be given in evidence. Do you understand?'

'What did he do?' the man's wife squealed, but her query was interrupted by her husband's caged-animal roar.

'What the fuck? No, you can't arrest me. I haven't done anything.'

He turned to me.

'You can fuck off,' he said.

He turned to Pete. 'You can fuck off.'

Finally, he turned to Sasha. 'And you, *especially*, can fuck off. Come on, Maggie, let's get the fuck out of here.'

He extended a hand towards his wife, meaning for her to take it, but Sasha was quick. She whipped her handcuffs out of her holder, and slapped one side of the cuffs on his wrist.

'You didn't seem to hear me, sir, but I am arresting you for intending to cause alarm and distress, and for using a racial slur against this gentleman here,' Sasha said.

It's admirable that Sasha was able to get a cuff on him so quickly. I've seen her deal with prisoners very elegantly before – but there was no way she was going to be able to hold this ample-sized, gelatinous mess of misplaced anger by herself.

'Pete, get some backup and a caged van,' I said. He took half a step back to get outside of the angry man's range, and reached for his radio immediately. The man pointed at me.

'Are you in charge here? What happened to my rights, eh? I know my fucking rights. You can't arrest me. You don't have a fucking warrant. This is fucking kidnapping.'

As he was jabbing his finger half-heartedly in the direction of my eyes, I saw my chance. Keeping eye contact, I snuck my right hand to my handcuffs, took them out of the holster, and attached them to the hand that was pointing into my face.

We use Hiatt Speedcuffs, which are handcuffs with bars between the two cuffs, instead of a chain. They're bulkier than the cuffs you tend to see police officers in cop shows carry around, but they do have a huge advantage: once you have one cuff attached to your prisoner, you can use the cuffs for leverage. Dubbed 'pain compliance' by the training team at Hendon, with these cuffs if it looks as though you're liable to lose control of a prisoner, you can use the stiff bar to manipulate them to do what you want.

'Place your hands behind your back, sir, and I will explain everything to you.'

'Fuck you,' he said once again, without showing any inclination to pay heed to my suggestion.

'Sir, you do understand that swearing at me isn't going to do you any good, right?' I said.

'What the fuck are you going to do? Isn't this a fucking free country? I know my rights, and you've got no fucking reason for fucking kidnapping me! Now let me get the fuck out of these hand-fucking-cuffs, before I fuck you up.' Clearly my strategy to get him to swear less was less than efficient.

'Sir, are you threatening me?' I asked, as light-heartedly as I could.

'Fucking right I am. I'll fuck you up, you little bastard. What are you gonna do? Shout at me a little? You're not the police. You haven't even got a fucking gun, you gutless pussy.'

'My friend, you see this little badge here?' I said, and pointed at the name badge on my Metvest. 'You see where it says Police Constable? And here's my identification.' I whipped out my warrant card with one hand, as I was still holding on to the cuff that was holding his right hand. 'Can you see the bit where it says "Warrant"? That's all the warrant I need to arrest you. I assure you all three of us are police officers. You're going to get arrested now, and we'll have a chat about all of this at the station.'

Unappeased, the man suddenly moved both his hands up at high speed. I only just managed to hold on to the cuff on my side, but Sasha's slipped out of her hand. The spare metal cuff glanced her across her face, and sent her glasses flying. She yelped in pain, but recomposed herself quickly. She took one step on to one of the chairs behind the man, then another to get on to the table. Through her swift climbing-on-the-table action, she was suddenly tall enough to reach the cuff. She jumped, grabbed the cuff, and came crashing back to the ground, taking the man's arm with her.

'Place your arms behind your back now,' I said. As the word 'now' passed my lips, I twisted the cuffs towards his back. In training, this is a move we practise on each other all the time – you'll have to take my word for this; a sharply twisted set of handcuffs is powerful tool for persuasion.

During this, Pete had finished his radio call, and approached the man's wife. Flashing her a charm-buster of a smile, he had firmly guided her away from the struggle in progress.

Sasha and I somehow managed to get the man's hands behind his back at the same time, and we connected the two empty cuffs together behind his back. With Sasha's cuff holding his left hand, my cuff holding his right, and both sets of cuffs attached to each other, we finally had the man under control.

A small crowd had gathered around us, which Pete was in the middle of placating.

'Let's just step over this way,' Sasha said, and pointed towards the awkwardly-shaped short leg of the L in an attempt to at least get this guy a little bit out of the way, away from the other guests in the restaurant.

To my surprise, the American went along with the command, but of course not without making a protest.

'I have my First Amendment rights,' the man shouted. 'You can't tell me what I can say and what I can't say! You'll hear from my embassy, you fucking Nazis! This is the last time I'll visit your stinking little island! Fuck you, get off me,' he screamed, as he struggled against the two sets of handcuffs.

It wasn't a pretty sight.

'I have the right to free speech! I didn't punch anybody; I didn't steal anything. Why the fuck am I wearing these handcuffs?' he said, before reiterating, like a tediously skipping record, that he knew his rights.

'Right, let me explain this to you,' I started. 'Your First Amendment doesn't apply here—'

'Fuck you. Like hell my First Amendment doesn't apply,' he shouted at the top of his considerable lung capacity and vocal volume. 'Have you ever heard of the fucking Constitution? I want my lawyer. Why didn't you offer me a lawyer? That's one of my fucking rights, you know!'

'Mate, I don't care what you think your rights are,' I exploded. I had had it with this guy; nothing pisses me off more than people who 'know their rights' after having watched one too many American cop shows. 'You have the right to a solicitor, but not until we make it back to the police station. In the meantime, do you remember the bit Sasha here told you about "you do not have to say anything"? That's basically the same as "your right to remain silent", and I suggest you use it.'

He half-grunted, half-snorted, which I choose to interpret as: 'My good sir, I do apologise for causing you such an inconvenience, and I would relish in silently listening to you for the foreseeable future.'

'So, your First Amendment is part of the Bill of Rights. I appreciate that piece of legislation, but you are in the UK, and the First Amendment – along with the rest of the US Constitution – is part of US law. It does not apply here.'

'But I'm an American citizen—'

'When I am in the US, I have to adhere to US law,' I interjected.

'When I'm here, I have to stick to local laws. The same goes for you, when you're in England you're bound by English law. I don't know how you normally speak to people in the US, but in the UK, we've got a piece of legislation known as the Public Order Act.

'The POA is a set of laws that was designed to make England a nicer place. At its most serious, in section 1, it covers riots. At its least serious, it covers people wandering around in the streets yelling obscenities.

'Do you recall what you said to the security guard earlier? A word starting with an N?' I enquired.

'Yeah. When someone is being a fucking nigger, I'll call them a nigger,' the man grunted.

'Well, there's a problem with that: your freedom of speech does not extend to swearing at random strangers, especially if you use racial slurs,' I explained. 'That's a pretty serious matter, and I won't stand for it. It's bad enough that you were swearing at me and my colleagues, but swearing at the cashier and calling the security guy, who was only trying to help sort things out, what you did is not appropriate.'

I was about to explain in further depth exactly how much trouble he was in, when I spotted Pete waving at me to come over. I looked over at Sasha. She shrugged. 'I got this,' she said, and took a firmer grip of the man's handcuff.

I believed her, and walked over to Pete.

'Just got off the radio,' he started. 'Something's kicked off in the next borough, and they've sent a load of support from our shift over there.'

'Keep an eye on our American friend over here,' I told Pete, and I walked over to the security guard.

'Hey, have you had a chance to look at the security tape?' I asked him.

'Yeah, he clearly handed over a tenner and a twenty. I guess he's just not used to the money over here,' he said, with a shrug. He didn't seem particularly upset.

'We've got a bit of a problem. I don't feel comfortable transporting this fellow on foot, and all the support is tied up on another incident in the next borough at the moment.' The security guard nodded; he understood where this was going. 'If I encourage him to calm down and apologise, would that be okay?'

'I'm not happy, man,' he said, and handed me Sasha's glasses; they came off during the struggle, and he must have picked them up.

'Thanks,' I said, inspecting the glasses. They seemed to be more or less in one piece.

'But yeah, if he apologises and gets the hell out of my shop, I'm happy. I'm not here to be abused, but I haven't got time for shit like this neither.'

'Yeah, I completely understand. I'm sorry about the lack of support, but our prisoner transport vans are deployed elsewhere. I'd much rather have taken him in, but apparently something serious is taking place, and I don't really know what it is.' I shrugged apologetically.

'No worries, I understand,' he said.

I went back to the American.

'Right, buddy, there's two ways we can do this. We can either sit here and wait for a van to arrive, check you into custody, interview you, and deal with you properly, or we can send you on your way. What would you prefer?' I asked.

'I get to choose?' he asked, clearly thinking I was trying to catch him out with some sort of practical joke.

'Well, yes. But if you just want to walk away, you're going to need to do some serious apologising, starting with my colleagues here, then with me and then the staff here,' I said.

'Could you please take these handcuffs off me,' he said. 'I would like to shake everyone's hands, and apologise properly.'

I wasn't too sure what to do about that particular request. If I am being honest, I knew it was more luck than skill that enabled us to get him in cuffs in the first place, and I wasn't sure we were going to be able to pull off the same stunt twice.

I conferred with Pete and Sasha. They were both sitting just behind the American. First I spotted Sasha; her face was completely red. Glancing over at Pete, I realised they were both shaking with laughter. Both of them were trying their best to keep the giggles under control, and I was getting pissed off. What the hell was going on?

'Are you okay to take the cuffs off?' I asked them. Pete opened his mouth, but didn't trust his voice not to break into all-out laughter, and so simply nodded, produced his handcuff keys and let the giant free from his captivity.

'So, about those apologies . . .' I said.

'Erm, yes. Of course, sir,' he said. As if struck with a magic wand, his behaviour had completely changed. He was as polite as they come.

Turning to Sasha first: 'I let anger get the better of me, ma'am. I am so very sorry. Please forgive me.'

Next to Pete, then to me with slight variations on the same apologetic theme.

With that out of the way, he bounded out to the main part of the restaurant, much faster than I would have expected from a man his size. I ran after him, but needn't have panicked; he was the very picture of grace and politeness. He tried to tip both of the restaurant staff £20 for their trouble and the offence caused. They refused to take his money, although they were happy to accept a spectacularly well-performed grovel of an apology.

Finally, he turned to me again, apologised once more, and whisked himself and his wife out of the restaurant.

I immediately rang in to cancel the van, and was asked by the operator to return to Mike Delta (the station identifier for our home police station).

'Yes, yes, received. We'll take the bus!' I radioed back.

'What the hell happened back there?' I asked, as I turned back into the area beside the counter to find Pete and Sasha collapsed on the floor, howling with laughter.

'He . . .' Sasha began, but had to abort her explanation attempt in favour of gasping for breath

'She . . .' Pete said, before being similarly overcome with giggles.

'Jesus,' I said, getting annoyed.

I decided to leave them to their fits of debilitating laughter, and I joined the restaurant staff to get confirmation in writing that they were happy that the case was resolved by the American apologising.

When we finally left the restaurant, my two colleagues had gathered their wits a little. A little, at least.

'What the . . .?' I asked.

'Well, when you went to speak to the security guard,' Pete said, 'the wife walked up to her husband, and said that if they had to stay here for another five minutes he wouldn't get any blow-jobs for the rest of the year.' The last part of his sentence was barely audible, as both he and Sasha were in fits of laughter again.

'Jeez,' I said, fighting to stop my inner eye from envisioning any sort of sexual encounter between the two of them. 'You are buying the beers at the end of this shift, Pete. I'm definitely going to need some mental bleach to get that picture out of my mind.'

Hell hath no fury like an 11-year-old without BBM

'We've just had report of criminal damage in progress, outside 12 Church Walk. An IC2[7] youth, around 11 years of age, smashing up a car. On an I-grade.'

On this shift, I was an Incident Response Vehicle (IRV) driver – meaning I was responding to emergency calls about incidences that had recently happened or were still taking place.

When we are on duty, we're assigned call signs comprised of two different radio-calling identifiers. One of them is our shoulder number (in my case, Mike Delta 592), which only changes if you are promoted to a different rank or you transfer to another borough. The other is the call sign of the vehicle or unit we are assigned to. This changes from day to day, although most call signs have particular duties; for example, one will be the Missing Persons car, another will be an 'odd jobs' car, and others will be assigned only to super-urgent calls.

My call sign for the radio that day was Mike Delta 20. Thus far, it had been a dreadfully slow day, so the call coming in over

[7] White or Hispanic person

the radio engaged me enough to stir myself me into some semblance of excitement. I don't mind chasing after a group of troublemaking kids for a few minutes if it wakes me up.

I reached for the PTT[8] lever in my car, and pushed it down.

'Show two-zero,' I spoke into the microphone mounted next to my sun visor, and heard a distorted version of my own voice, feeding back through the radio I had clipped to my Metvest.

'Received,' replied the operator above the echo.

I pressed the '999' button on my dash, and the car's mobile disco facilities sprang into life. As the siren wailed, I spun the car around. Church Walk was just around the corner. I careened around the last bend, the slightest hint of a squeal coming from my tyres against the asphalt, and saw a young chap climbing over a low fence.

He's not running away, I thought. *In fact, he's coming towards me.*

'Show TOA[9] for Mike Delta two-zero,' I said, as I engaged the 'run lock' and climbed out of the Vauxhall Astra.

Run lock is one of the fun features built into a police car. It enables us to press a button, take the keys and lock the car with the engine running. If anyone tries to put the car in gear or open a door, the engine stops again. Run lock is useful when you have to leave your car parked somewhere with the radio and the flashing lights still operating: by leaving the engine running, it doesn't run the battery flat, but nobody can steal the car either!

'Hi there. You okay?' I asked the kid, as he came towards me. He nodded.

'You haven't seen anyone trying to smash up a car, have you?' He nodded again.

'That was me,' he said, and shrugged with a lack of

---

[8] Push To Talk button: The button that opens a radio channel and enables me to transmit with my radio.

[9] Time Of Arrival

commitment that made me stop in my tracks. How do you make a motion showing a lack of caring without caring? Mentally, I was shaking my head at this kid's utter lack of . . . well . . . anything.

I blinked a couple of times.

'Uhm . . . okay. Why did you smash up a car? Where is it?' He pointed at a dark red Volvo that was parked outside number ten.

We walked over to the car together, just as another police car showed up.

'TOA two-six,' my radio crackled, as the two officers climbed out of the car and started wandering towards us. I was about to send them on their way again, when a man emerged from one of the houses. An extremely agitated man.

'He smash the car! He smash the car!' the man shouted in a Turkish accent. He was walking briskly, gesticulating wildly. I took another look at the Volvo. It could have done with a wash, for sure, but all the windows seemed to be intact, and I couldn't see any obvious damage.

'What did he do?' I asked the man, as I gave him a once-over. He was wearing a pair of tracksuit bottoms, a food-stained T-shirt and the air of someone who had just rolled out of bed.

'He smash the car!' he said again.

I glanced back and forth at my colleagues. We deal with traffic collisions on a daily basis. We have seen a lot of smashed cars in our time.

This, I concluded, was *not* a smashed car.

'In June! He smash the car!'

'What exactly did you tell the people when you called 999?' I asked him, as it dawned on me what was going on.

'I say he smash the car!'

'Sir,' I said, 'You can't dial 999 about an incident that happened several months ago. If someone is smashing up your car, breaking into your house, or attacking you, call 999. With this—' I sighed. Realising my approach was futile, I changed tack. 'Do you know this young man?' I asked him, as I pointed at the kid.

'Yes,' the man said. 'He is my son.'

'He stole my Blackberry!' the kid piped up.

I'll save you the confounding banality of reporting a running dialogue. It took us the best part of 40 minutes to complete the puzzle of what had happened – the kind of puzzle that sits on the shelf until the cat has taken off with half a dozen pieces, and nobody really cares whether it's ever completed or not anyway.

I would be lying if I said that my job didn't involve dealing with a lot of this type of puzzle.

It turned out that back in June the father had taken the son's Blackberry as punishment for something or other – as parents are wont to do. In my day, we were sent to our room right after dinner, or deprived of watching *Columbo* for an evening. These days, the kids have to give up their Blackberry privileges.

Fair enough.

The boy retaliated for this grave miscarriage of justice by taking a cricket bat to the family car, smashing up the bonnet, the windshield and a couple of the side windows. The police were called, and the kid was taken in for criminal damage.

This time, the little scoundrel had started a fight at school, and once again the dad took his mobile away. Then ensued a lot of screaming and ranting. The dad thought he was going to smash up the car again, so he called the police.

I'd heard enough. I took the boy aside.

'Mate, why do you do stuff like that?' I asked him. 'You can't go around starting fights and smashing up cars – that's not going to get you any friends. I understand you might get frustrated and angry, but you're a clever kid, and it's not good news if your own dad has to keep calling the police on you.'

The boy replied (I swear to god this isn't a word of a lie), 'I have anger-management issues.'

'Uhm . . . Who told you that?' I asked. 'Have you been to see a doctor?'

He hadn't. This was a 13-year-old kid who had self-diagnosed himself with anger-management issues. I didn't know what to make of any of it.

'He's in a gang, you know,' the kid suddenly said.

'Who?' I tried to clarify.

'My dad. He's in a gang.'

Over the past hour, I had already caught him out in half a dozen lies – was this another trick? As a precaution, I called Carl, one of my colleagues, over and asked him to run the father and the kid through the PNC[10], CAD, and Crimint[11] to check whether we had any intel[12] on them.

'What does he do?' I asked the boy, mostly just to keep him talking.

'He has a gun,' the kid replied, looking at the tips of his Converses as he spoke.

Carl was just getting off the radio. He came towards me, shrugged, and shook his head in a manner that I took to mean there was nothing particularly suspicious about either of them.

'A gun? Really? Where does he keep it?' I asked the kid.

'In his car, under where the spare wheel is,' he said, and glanced up at my face to gauge my reaction. 'I've seen it. It's black.'

Now, I was facing a choice. If there is a suspicion of guns, I can't really do anything without Trojan assistance – i.e. armed police – but the kid had been lying to me all morning, and he had already implied several bad things about his dad, apparently

---

[10] Police National Computer

[11] The Metropolitan Police-wide criminal intelligence database

[12] 'Intel' refers to Intelligence. Checking for intel usually just means that we check any previous calls and all the various databases we have available to see if we know anything about a place, person, or vehicle.

only to get back at him. At the same time, I couldn't ignore this piece of information, either. Since the dad indicated that the car was the suspected goal for the son's attack, it gave me an idea.

'Can I see your keys for a second?' I asked the dad. He dug the car keys out of his pocket, and as he did, I took a closer look at him. He didn't appear to have any clothing on him that could hide a firearm. I took the keys off him and turned back to Carl.

'The kid's just told me his dad has a gun in the car. Nick him for suspicion of possession of a section five firearm. Get Belinda to help you,' I told him.

Carl walked over to Belinda, said a few words, and together they approached the dad. They cuffed him with his hands behind his back before he had any idea of what was happening.

He was handcuffed in a 'back to back' configuration, creatively named such because the backs of your hands are facing each other, behind your back. Other ways of handcuffing people are a 'front stack' (imagine folding your arms, and having a set of rigid handcuffs applied from wrist to wrist), or a 'rear stack' (the same, but on your back). It's also *possible* to do a 'palm-to-palm', but since we use rigid handcuffs, if you're going to cuff someone palm-to-palm you may as well not bother handcuffing them at all. It doesn't do much to impede movement, and they could potentially use the rigid bar between the cuffs as a weapon.

The dad started struggling, shouting abuse at my colleagues whilst they searched him, but they didn't find anything untoward. I kept an eye on them, just to make sure everything was okay, but Belinda and Carl seemed to have the situation under control.

I started walking over to the Volvo, but the kid stopped me.

'Not that one! That one,' he said, pointing towards a Mazda MX-5 parked further up the road.

I was rather doubtful at this point; I have *owned* an MX-5. They are great fun – proper little drivers' cars – but there's one thing they don't have, and that's a spare wheel. I take a look at the key ring the dad gave me but, unsurprisingly, the keys he gave me for the Volvo were Volvo keys. There weren't any keys that would fit on the Mazda on the key ring.

'Do you know where the keys are?' I asked the boy.

'Yeah,' he said, and sprinted off. Two seconds later, he came running back out of the house, clutching a set of keys.

I opened the MX-5's boot. There were a couple of holdalls in there, but they were empty. I was pissed off with the kid – lying about a gun in your father's car? In my head, I was already formulating the stern 'talking to' I was going to give him; already envisioning the grovelling I would have to do to the dad after arresting him for no reason whatsoever. Images of formal complaints, and of me having to explain myself to the borough commander, flickered through my brain.

This was going to be a long day.

On a whim, partly to buy time before apologising to the Dad, I lifted up the floor carpet . . . and I noticed something. The whole carpet in the boot was raised up on a block of carefully cut Styrofoam. It was incredibly well done, and the minor alteration to the car boot raised the boot floor by just an inch or so. It was nearly invisible. The Styrofoam was clad in a thin layer of fabric, and there was a hole cut in the material. I could see a small loop of material, so I carefully manipulated it with the tip of my biro, lifting it up, ever so slowly.

Bingo. There *was* a gun in there. A Glock, perhaps? I didn't know for certain – I'm not great with firearms.

I pushed the flap shut with the tip of my pen, moved the floor carpet back into place and closed the boot, locking the car up carefully. I walked over to the father, and gave a nod to Belinda.

'It's a gun,' I said. She arrested him for possession, and I got on the radio.

'Mike Delta receiving five-nine-two,' I transmitted.

'Five-nine-two, go ahead.'

'I'm going to need Trojan assistance. We found a gun in the boot of a car,' I said.

'Oh, and could you send a van on the hurry-up, please, I don't know if anyone is watching us. We've also got a kid we're going to have to take into custody.'

Every damn time I complain – even if it's just in my head – that a shift is too quiet, something ridiculous happens.

I suppose this is why we generally use the acronym QT – in order to avoid saying 'Quiet Time'.

In this instance, we were on the scene for another ten hours.

My colleagues returned to the nick[13], taking with them the father and son duo, along with a further five officers who had to come out to do a section 18 search of the dad's house. We found another two handguns, a rifle, a small amount of class-A drugs and a sizeable stash of ammunition for the weapons in the house. We also found another handgun carefully taped under the passenger seat, in another hollow cut into the upholstery of the MX-5. It turned out that the dad wasn't an active gang member, but that the local gangs used him as a handler, to make sure their guns weren't found during raids on the houses of known gang members.

I guess if there's anything to learn from this, it is: don't take your kid's Blackberry away from him if you've got a gun in the back of your car. And if you do, don't call the police on him yourself.

Or, you know, don't hold weapons for gang members. That might be even easier.

---

[13] 'The nick' is slang for your home police station – or the closest police station with custody cells.

A pinprick is nothing like a paper cut

'GET BACK!' I screamed at the top of my lungs, as I slowly shuffled away from the man standing opposite me on the seventh-floor
landing of a council estate.

The staircase I had just ascended was behind me. To the right
of me, there was a low black railing and a 70-foot drop. In front of
me was a Customer[14].

The man seemed dazed, not entirely with it in general, and
absolutely, feather-spittingly furious.

Something had happened to him. He had completely lost the
Ordinance Survey maps and headed out into the deepest, worst-
lit corners of incoherence. He was sobbing, shouting, mumbling,
drooling, spitting. The words 'Elise' and 'I'm going to fucking kill
him' kept being repeated.

My adrenaline boost was giving me tunnel vision and aural
exclusion. I was aware of it, but I wasn't able to use it: I couldn't
hear or see anything apart from the man I was facing. He wasn't
a very tall man – about five foot seven, perhaps. He was around

---

[14] The Metropolitan Police is so 'customer-focused' these days that everyone we
deal with is semi-sarcastically referred to as a 'customer', even if they are caught
red-handed, halfway into someone's bedroom window during a burglary.

40 years old, IC1, with a build that suggested a long, hard life of substance abuse. He was hunched forward, holding onto the railing with his left hand.

I reached for my radio and pressed *the* button – the orange one, right between the volume dial and the stubby antenna on my Motorola personal radio. Officially, it's known as the Emergency Assistance Button. Frequently, it's known as the 'whoops' or the 'shit has hit the fan button' too. In this case, it was the 'I need some bloody backup, bloody quickly' button.

As I pressed down, the other transmission that was in progress (something about an RTC[15]) was cancelled, and I could speak for ten seconds without having to clutch my radio's transmit button.

'Urgent assistance required,' I said, as calmly as I could, without breaking eye contact with the man, who was edging closer to me very slowly. I told the radio where I was, and followed up with the words that I knew would catch everyone's attention: 'IC1 male with a knife.'

I took a firmer grip of the GFLB[16] I had in my right hand, and crept back until I felt my foot touch something behind me. I realised with a jolt that the only direction I *really* wanted to go – further away from the addict in front of me – was blocked by a wall.

The man didn't have an actual knife. 'Knife' is what you say over the radio to convey 'sharp weapon'. Samurai sword? *Knife.* Bayonet? *Knife.* Stanley blade? *Knife.* Surgeon's scalpel? *Knife.* Similarly, all bat-like weapons are 'sticks', and any projectile weapon is a 'gun'. If that sounds a little bit backwards, well, I'd urge you not to worry about it too much. When you are dosed to the eyelids with adrenaline in an extreme situation, it's a lot easier to say 'knife' than trying to decide whether you're facing a madman with

---

[15] Road Traffic Collision
[16] Gravity Friction-Lock Baton

a *foil*, a *sabre* or an *épée*. From our point of view, if it cuts, slashes or stabs, it's a knife.

This particular madman, however, was holding a whole different class of 'knife'. In his hand he had an injection needle of some sort. It was tiny. The only reason I knew he was clutching it was the occasional flash of surgical steel in the overhead lighting.

I've faced suspects with a baffling array of weapons. Guns, of course. Bats, knives, tyre irons, rolling pins, cast-iron pans, and even a chainsaw once. Nothing scares me as much as a hypodermic needle. When you're against somebody with a bat, it's a fair fight: they have a stick, you have a stick, you both have a bit of a tussle, they get arrested, job done. You may walk away with some bruises, perhaps even a broken bone, but ultimately it's a situation you've been trained to handle. Guns are slightly worse, of course, but there's a solution for that too, and over my years in the Metropolitan Police, I've perfected the art of running-away-very-fast-and-waiting-for-the-cavalry-to-arrive.

When faced with a needle, you have a huge problem: if they come close enough to be wrestled to the ground and arrested, they're close enough to give you a tiny scratch. It seems strange to be completely out of your head on adrenaline because of a weapon you can barely see, and yet a million statistics back you up. For example, in England, injecting drugs causes 90 per cent of all cases of hepatitis C and 6 per cent of all HIV cases. I've had my hepatitis jabs, of course, but a cure for HIV is still far enough away that I'd rather not have to deal with it.

The man took a step closer just as my radio jumped back into life. 'Mike Delta five-nine-two. Status update?' I briefly touched my PTT[17].

'Could do with some help here, guys. He's armed with a hypodermic needle.'

[17] Push To Talk

'Received. ETA one minute,' the operator fired back.

I tried talking to the man again, interrupting his incoherent tirade: 'Mate, let's get you some help. We'll find out what's happening, and I'll help you. I promise.'

He took a step closer still, but some of the wildness seemed to have been extinguished from his eyes; a sign that I was getting through to him, I hoped.

'Mate, I know you're hurting. I can help you. I don't want anyone to get hurt,' I said, and involuntarily moved my baton side to side a little. My knuckles were white from gripping my 21 inches of extendable stainless steel. The movement caught his eye. He straightened up slightly and, in the process, slumped lightly against the railing.

Behind him, I spotted two of my colleagues. They must have gone up the wrong stairway into the estate and ended up behind the man. Or perhaps they knew the layout better, and went around on purpose?

Whatever the reason, they held an advantage by being behind him and it suddenly became my job to *keep* that advantage. I started talking, careful not to stop. I knew that I had to keep his attention on me.

'What's your name? Can I call you Simon?' This is an old trick of psychology: call someone by the wrong name, and they will be rattled enough to give up their real name.

'Matthew,' he barked back.

'Matthew? That's great. My name is Matthew too. We're like brothers, you and I. You're not that much older than me. Perhaps you could have been my bigger brother, and we could have been Matthew and Matthew. That would have been confusing, wouldn't it?' I forced a laugh. Matthew looked confused; he started to laugh, but then remembered whatever it was that was bothering him in the first place, and a look of determination came over his face.

My colleagues advanced behind him. Our tactics worked. Matthew was oblivious to the impending attack. Craig grabbed his arm and Tim put him in a headlock.

'Drop the needle,' Tim shouted.

Immediately Matthew did as he was told. For a brief moment I thought he might try to throw himself off the balcony, but the three of us held him back, and minutes later he was led downstairs in handcuffs.

When we finally had Matthew under arrest, we ran him through the PNC. His PNC record had warnings for drugs, violence and for being a known carrier of hepatitis A and C.

The three of us looked at each other, and a shiver ran down my spine.

'I'll take a knife fight over this any day of the week,' I half joked. Instead of laughing, my colleagues nodded silently in agreement.

We had all walked a little bit closer to the edge than we were comfortable with.

Sudden Death

My Ticket had expired.

The *ticket* I'm referring to is my police driving licence. As well as a standard DVLA driving licence, in order to be allowed to drive any police vehicle, you need to have a special driving licence. To receive this licence, officers do a course, followed by theoretical and practical exams.

Police driving licences come in different levels, starting at 'level 4'. This is the 'boring' ticket that allows you to drive from one place to another, but not on blues and twos[18]. You can do a 'compliant stop' – which means that you can drive behind somebody and turn your blue lights on to pull them over – but if they drive off, you have to call off the pursuit. This happened to me once when I had only the basic ticket, and I felt pretty daft having to let the guy drive away. Thankfully, in London there's never a helicopter far off. The helicopter followed him to a petrol station, where I was able to go and arrest them. It transpired that he had a sizeable amount of drugs in the

---

[18] 'Blues' are the flashing blue lights. 'Twos' refer to the two-tone sirens used on police cars (the ones that kids normally ape when they run around the house shouting 'neeh-naah-neeh-naah').

car. 'Sorry, I didn't see you, officer,' the driver had said. Nice touch.

There are dozens of different driving courses you can take. I have a solo ticket (that's for riding police motorbikes) and the advanced driving qualification. The advanced course is rather interesting, and includes all sorts of high-speed pursuit stuff. It's a shame that my end of the borough has 40mph limits (or less) everywhere, so I never get to open the cars up properly.

Much like normal driving licences, police licences expire. Unlike normal driving licences, they expire rather quickly. When I'd realised mine was almost up, I'd gone to the driving school at Hendon to have it renewed, but the instructor I was meant to go out with had had to break his appointment when he was called off to something or other. You'd be surprised how often that sort of thing happens; I have a feeling he moonlights for the DPG[19], which would explain a lot.

An expired ticket isn't a disaster. It normally means you end up 'operating' on a Panda – a term still in use despite police patrol cars having not been black and white for several decades – or one of the area cars, with someone else driving. However, on one occasion, I also managed to make it to work late. As a punishment the skipper[20] decided to send me out on foot patrols through some of the shopping centres and markets that had recently been plagued with drugs and shoplifting.

Whilst assigning the job, the skipper explained it would 'help build character'. I had pretended to be insulted and grumpy as I left. 'Pretended' because, honestly, I don't really mind foot patrols all that much. It does mean you're not on response duties, but it's actually quite nice to have an opportunity to stroll around the

[19] Diplomatic Protection Group
[20] Slang for sergeant

borough for a day. You talk to people, you get some exercise, and it's a completely different experience to spending all day flying, tyres a-screeching, from call to call.

The morning's foot patrol, however, had turned out to be less than pleasant. Heavy clouds were sagging with the weight of grey depression, ready to ejaculate their heavy, sleety load all over my freshly washed overcoat. January will always be a dreadful time to be on foot patrol.

Thankfully, I'd managed to spend a fair bit of time getting to know the café owners around my sector of the borough. A chat and a coffee here, a quick vandalism report and a cup of tea there – it all makes the world spin merrily on.

Lunchtime came along eventually and, since it was a Friday, I decided to treat myself to a greasy delicacy from Burger King.

Just as I finished the last bite of my double whopper, my radio interrupted my daydreaming.

'Five-nine-two receiving Mike Delta?' it squawked.

'Retheifsglowblead,' I replied, with my mouth full of burger and my last two fries.

The couple sitting on the next table glanced over momentarily, before hunching over their trays, laughing so hard I briefly thought they might do themselves an injury.

'You broke up there, say again?'

'Receiving, go ahead!' I repeated, smiling at the couple, with a shrug. I ended my transmission.

'Hey, they don't like waiting, what can I say?' I said to the giggling couple, and winked.

'We have a Code Zulu up on Eastern Terrace. Are you free to deal?' the CAD operator asked.

It has been a long time since you were able to buy an off-the-shelf 'police scanner' to listen in on police conversations, like they do in the movies, but there remains a rather obvious security flaw:

as I sit there, finishing my lunch, the couple at the table next to mine will be able to overhear everything my colleagues talk about. Mostly, it will be boring stuff: a shoplifter, a colleague needing an Op Reclaim recovery of an uninsured car, or CCTV reporting some youths drinking in the park. However, occasionally, much more serious matters will be transmitted over radio.

As a precaution, our Airwave radios are encrypted. Not as heavily as elsewhere, though. On American cop shows, you often hear them say things like '10-4' (we'd say, 'Received'), '10-23' (we say, 'Stand by, please') or '417A' (we say, 'Suspect with a knife'). You don't really want to have to look up all sorts of inane codes for every thinkable situation (apparently '10-41' means 'Will you be requiring an ambulance?' What's wrong with saying, '*Will you be requiring an ambulance?*'). However, in the UK we do have a few codes that we use, even over the military-grade-encrypted radios. We'd use a code like 'Code X-ray' for a sexual assault, for example; 'Code Yankee' could be a bomb threat.

The situation the operator was asking me to attend was a Code Zulu – a Sudden Death.

Sudden Deaths are the bread-and-butter of policing; whenever a 'sudden death' happens, police are called as a matter of course. I'm actually a little bit fuzzy on what defines a 'sudden death', but I believe it is any death that doesn't happen as the cause of an obvious accident, and to someone who has not seen a doctor in a couple of weeks.

'A few weeks? Oh my, I haven't been to my GP in over a year,' you might say. That was certainly my reaction when I first found out what a sudden death was. However, the two-week rule means that anybody who has had recent medical issues – heart attacks, late-stage cancer and so on – isn't automatically classed as 'sudden', because, well, they're not technically sudden.

As a police officer, I sometimes fear I have become a little bit blasé about death. I see dead bodies relatively routinely as part of my job. Whether a person expires through a traffic accident, work accident, suicide or violence, they will end up across our desks sooner or later, and as a response copper, I'm sent to deal with all of it first-hand.

Sudden deaths are always eerie, though, because they are unexpected. I suppose being side-swiped by a lorry is also unexpected, but at least there's something oddly honest about a traffic death. One particularly memorable sudden death I attended was at a cinema. We had received a call from a very distressed cinema manager. Apparently, a 25-year-old girl had bought a ticket to a matinee showing and quietly sat down in one of the back rows of the cinema, where she remained seated until the credits had finished. The cleaners poked her to wake her up, and she flopped over, dead as last week's kebab dinner. At first, we thought she was a suicide case (either that, or she simply lost her will to live halfway through M. Night Shyamalan's *The Happening*, which, to be fair, is a conclusion any coroner worth their salt would accept). However, it turned out that she had had an obscure type of heart failure.

Today's case was at a residential property a short distance from me.

'Yeah, I'm free. I'm on foot, but I'll stroll over. I'll be about ten minutes,' I responded (much sooner than the length of the digressing monologue above would indicate).

'Great. Please liaise with thirty-four and seventy-one, they are en route,' the CAD operator concluded. I slowed my pace a little. No point in getting to the party early.

Just as I walked through the front doorway of the property, Jeff, one of the newer members on our team, burst out of the living room and launched himself full-speed into the toilet. I suppressed a giggle. I could hear him throwing up his lunch as

I walked towards the living room. I noticed immediately that the house was in absolutely meticulous condition. Every photograph was so perfectly straight that I suspected the owner had used a spirit level. The carpets looked crisply shampooed, the windows were spotless; apart from an incredible swarm of flies, the house was practically a model home. It was a far cry from some of the crack dens we have to wade around, some of which are so bad you feel obliged to wipe your boots on the doormat on the way *out* of the flat, so that you don't make the street dirty when you leave.

I turned the corner into the living room, and the sight that met me was, put simply, grim. A man, who must have been quite obese, had died sitting on a chair in his living room. As he'd drawn his last breath, he'd fallen from his seat, and his ample body had come to rest against the radiator. Of course, seeing as it was January – and a pretty nippy January at that – the radiator had been at full blast.

The combination of the radiator heat and the dead body was not a good thing: the man had probably only been dead for about a week, but the warmth meant that the flies had bred much faster.

I am not sure what in particular had made Jeff bolt from the room to the bathroom. It could have been the sight of the maggots boring their way through the skin on the man's face and neck. It could have been the large stains where his gas-bloated skin had burst, spilling flies, maggots and bodily fluids on the carpet. My money would have been on the smell, though. The aroma of somebody who has been dead for a couple of weeks is something that stays with you for days. It is such a distinctive, persistent and piercing stench that I swear I can smell it now as I type this – even though I haven't had the misfortune of attending a sudden death in weeks.

'You all right, Matt?' I heard a weak voice behind me. It was Jeff.

'Yeah, bud. You feeling better?' I asked

'Man . . . I can just never get used to seeing people like that.'

'You will, eventually. Trust me. Who called it in?' I asked.

'A neighbour smelled him this morning, and called the landlord to complain, of all people.'

'Hah, the landlord, eh? You'd have thought people would have the sense to call *us*.'

'I spoke to the neighbour. He was in a state of complete shock,' Jeff said. 'He apologised so many times I thought for a moment he might have killed the guy himself. Turns out he's never seen a dead body before; he thought it was the smell of cat litter. The complaint to the landlord was about his neighbour having pets!'

I shuddered at the mention of furry little felines. The funny, cute videos on YouTube are only half the story: sure, cats are cute enough, but they're also vicious little carnivores. I've attended a sudden death where a pair of cats were in the house when their owner died. Suffice to say, the cats did not go hungry despite not being fed.

'Who would have known, eh?' I said.

'Yeah,' Jeff said, still standing at the door, looking at the bloated body slumped against the radiator. 'So . . . er . . . what do you reckon?'

'No idea, mate. He doesn't look that old,' I said. 'How did you get into the flat?'

'We had to kick the door in,' Jeff replied. 'Landlord couldn't get in; the latch was on.'

'Clearly, nobody killed the poor sod, so whatever he died of, it's probably nothing criminal. Best get him ready for the coroner, though, eh?'

Jeff excused himself and ran off to throw up some more. By now, I wasn't feeling too hot either.

Preparing someone for the coroner includes checking all the

property of the deceased – including their pockets. I could tell that this particular pockets-check was going to be unpleasant.

When Jeff returned, one of the sergeants was with him.

'What have we got, Delito?' the sergeant barked.

It was Mike Delta 71 – only ever known as 71. I'm sure he must *have* a name, and I'm sure his name is printed directly underneath 'Police Sergeant' on the Velcro nametag on his Metvest, but nobody ever uses it. I had made a dreadful mistake in the station café a few months before by doing my impersonation of 71's wife, as she, in the throes of carnal enlightenment, screams out 'Oh! Ooh! My god! Yes! seventy-one ! I'm coming! Coming so hard! Your truncheon is making me come! Sevent—' and that, ladies and gentlemen, is of course the precise moment when 71 walked into the café.

We haven't really been on speaking terms since.

I explained the goings-on so far, and 71 nodded in response. Meanwhile, Jeff had ducked away from the door again, except this time it was to laugh, not to throw up. He was one of the people who had cheered on my impersonation of Mrs 71.

'Jeff,' 71 barked. 'Come help Delito with this body.'

We had to place Mr Bloggs on his back in order to search him properly. Once we'd both put on gloves, Jeff moved the chair out of the way and took the body under one arm, whilst I picked up his other arm.

'Onto his back,' I said. 'Slowly. One . . . Two . . .'

We moved him on three, but the side of his head seemed to stick to the radiator. I watched the skin of his face stretch, ever so slowly, until finally it gave way. The dead man's head flopped back with a crunch. My eyes were glued to the radiator, where a disturbingly large amount of cheek skin was still sticking to the metal. Jeff let go of his side and leapt from the room. I dropped my side of the body as well, and the man hit the carpet with a thud.

The combination of the cheek stuck on the radiator and the sound of Jeff retching pushed me over the edge. I moved towards the doorway, but found my way blocked by Jeff, who had thrown up on 71's leg. I decided to take my hat off, and leave my lunch in it instead. I should have known Burger King would be a bad idea.

Bringing them back from the dead

Usually, we find out about traffic incidents over the radio. Either someone dials 999, or CCTV cameras pick up weird traffic movements and discover that two finely engineered boxes of iron and plastic have reduced each other to a set of insurance claims, and their drivers and passengers to 'casualties'.

However, I once drove by the scene of one accident just as it happened. My friend Kim, who also happened to be my operator that day, and I had just finished with an incredibly grievous case of a sudden death caused by a drugs overdose. As I pulled out of a junction, a motorcyclist who had been thrown from his bike came skidding past us.

We immediately stopped our car – blue lights blazing – using it to block the road, and got out to see what had happened.

'He's not breathing,' Kim said, once she had run over to him and flipped his visor open. 'I don't think he's breathing!'

I checked the road quickly; our vehicle was holding back any traffic from coming our way, which would have to do in terms of protecting us.

To be able to do fully effective CPR[21], you usually also need to

---

[21] CPR is short for Cardiopulmonary resuscitation; it's also known as 'heart massaging' or 'chest compressions'.

be able to give rescue breaths. To do that, you need access to the patient's mouth, and you'll be unsurprised to hear that a full-face motorcycle helmet doesn't really help in that respect.

It is commonly believed that you should never remove a motor-cyclist's helmet if he's been in an accident. As a general rule, that is true; motorcycle accidents have a high rate of spinal and head injuries, and removing the helmet can cause further injury to the spinal column. However, in many cases, you don't have the luxury of a choice: if someone stops breathing they have, at most, four minutes before they start suffering brain damage. They need CPR, which means the helmet has to come off – *pronto*.

I quickly got on my radio to get some more help.

'Mike Delta receiving?'

'Go ahead.'

'I need LAS on the hurry-up. IC1 male, aged around forty, has come off a motorbike. He's not breathing or responding, but no obvious injuries. No other casualties.'

'Received. LAS on the way. What's his status?'

'Not sure, we're starting ELS[22] now!' I barked back and cut the line. A bit rude, perhaps, but I didn't really have time for chit-chatting with the radio operator.

An ambulance was on its way, which meant that we would only have to deal with this fellow on our own for about 15 minutes at most.

Kim and I started the painfully slow process of taking his helmet off. We undid the chinstrap (which was a goddamn double-D clasp; great for motorcyclists, but a royal pain for rescue personnel). I stuck my hands into the helmet – one hand on each side of his neck, as far into the helmet as I could get – to steady his head. Kim, swearing under her breath, was gently rocking the helmet

---

[22] Emergency Life Support

back and forth, to very carefully get it off him. All the while, the motorcyclist didn't move a muscle.

After what felt like an eternity, we finally managed to remove his helmet. Kim produced a CPR mask out of nowhere – I had no idea she carried one around with her – and started performing rescue breaths as I unzipped the motorcyclist's jacket, ready to perform chest compressions.

Once he had had his rescue breaths, I started the compressions. The first push gave a horrible crunching sound. Here's something they don't often tell you in the first aid course: if you're doing CPR correctly, you're more than likely to break their sternum and ribs in the process. The first time it happened to me, I was so surprised and sickened that I dry-heaved. I was lucky not to throw up all over my own arms and my victim, but to my credit I didn't stop giving CPR.

With this particular patient, we only made it through two cycles before the ambulance arrived. They had an AED[23] on them, and started hooking the man up right away.

'Shock advised,' the AED machine bleated out.

'Stand clear,' one of the paramedics said, glancing around quickly to make sure no one was touching the patient, before pressing the button on the AED.

'Shock delivered,' an unnaturally calm voice spoke from the AED machine.

Almost immediately, our motorcyclist shot back to life. The change was rapid, and downright incredible. From the increasingly white colour he had had in the minutes since we'd found him, his face and lips turned instantly red, as he groaned and gasped for air.

---

[23] Automatic External Defibrillator. It's like those paddles they use in hospitals to 'shock' patients back to life, except more suitable for carrying around with you in an ambulance.

I too felt a rush of blood run to my ears, face and fingertips. It was almost as though my heart had decided to stop beating in sympathy with the motorcyclist's.

It is a rare thing to see someone brought back from the dead, and the feeling when it happens is indescribable.

And that, ladies and gentlemen, is one of the reasons why I absolutely love my job.

With the motorcyclist's chances looking a little bit better, I let my mind wander back to the accident. I was puzzled about what may have happened to the motorcyclist: the road was clear and dry, the visibility was good, it was early afternoon so there wasn't a lot of traffic around, and no one else appeared to have been involved. I looked at the bike, and other than the damage of the accident itself, I couldn't really see anything obviously wrong with it.

After hooking the man up to another one of their machines (I'm not a medic, so you'll have to forgive the vague terms – it was a machine that went 'beep' a lot), one of the paramedics provided a solution to the mystery.

'This guy has just had a heart attack,' he said, looking at the readouts on the little display. 'We'll take him with us, he's going to need to be looked after, but I think he'll be fine.'

As the paramedics loaded the motorcyclist into the back of their ambulance, the Traffic Police arrived to do an investigation. Traffic are usually called if there's a risk a collision is 'life changing or life threatening'. It didn't take long before they concurred with my initial assessment: nothing was wrong with the road or the bike. There was no sign that he even tried to hit the brakes – he just tumbled off the side of the motorcycle at about 30mph.

'Seems like the LAS guys were right,' the traffic copper said. 'Heart attack makes sense.'

The man was conveyed to hospital at full speed. Later we discovered he had a broken shin, a gallery of bruises and his very own, very first heart attack, but he did walk (well, hobble) out a few days later.

So . . . you're saying you were attacked by a ninja?

'Umm, I don't really know how to put this, officer. Last night I was walking up the street with my Xbox 360, and then a ninja came and punched me in the face. He stole my Xbox!'

'Why were you walking around with an Xbox on a Friday night?'

The fellow was about 15 seconds into his statement and already the officer taking the statement was desperately wishing he'd stayed in the café for another five minutes, just so he wouldn't have had to deal with this particular madman.

'Well, I was coming home from a company Christmas party. I was dressed in my gi.'

'What's a gi?'

'It's a suit. Kind of like pyjamas. You wear them in a dojo when you're competing in judo.'

'Do you do judo?'

'No.'

'So . . .'

'Well, I used to do judo. I used to be pretty good, actually.'

'Right, well, please do start from the beginning. Why were you wearing a judo suit on a Friday night?'

'Well, it was a costume party. As I said, the company Christmas do, so I wore my gi.'

'Right. And the Xbox?' the officer said, rapidly approaching the end of his tether.

If you draw the short straw at the beginning of your shift, you probably end up manning the front office – this is where MOPs[24] come in person to report incidents to the police. I'm not a huge fan of that job, for obvious reasons. The front office attracts a rather peculiar clientele – and I don't think I'm exaggerating by saying that at least a dozen people a few pennies short of a pound come through the front office every week. It's not all bad; at least you are warm, and you don't have to do a lot of running.

You just have to deal with a lot of *nutters*.

I hear you thinking: 'So, apart from clearly being "a bit nuts", what was so special about this particular fellow who had been attacked by a ninja?'

Well, he was *me*, before I became a police officer.

Maybe I should go back to the beginning . . .

I was working for a large company at the time, and we were having our annual Christmas party. As usual, there was a theme, and this time – thanks to a large deal that had been secured about a month earlier – the theme was Asia. There was a fancy-dress element, but – as per usual – I hadn't got around to doing anything for it.

The day before the party, a couple of my mates from the office discussed dressing up as kung-fu heroes. One of them had bought a bright yellow tracksuit and intended to go as Bruce Lee. In a moment of inspiration, I formed a plan: I would dust off my old martial arts gi, and go as a judoka.

It was immediately obvious to me that this was a

[24] Members of the Public

54

plan so brilliant it outshone a thousand suns: it was tenaciously Asia-related, and carried the additional bonus of me not having to actually *do* or *buy* anything – I could simply throw the gi on, and then go to the party. Score.

I made a point of shaving my head that morning, just to look extra 'ard, and went to the office as usual. I had a couple of comments about looking like a skinhead, but I shrugged them off; I'd been called worse in the office. At the end of the day, I went to a quick dinner at the local sushi restaurant (we were committed to the theme) with a couple of colleagues, before changing into my judo gi in the loos and heading to the party.

I'll spare you the details of the party itself. Suffice to say that there was an open bar, and my colleagues and I were damned if we were going to let a single drop of booze go to waste. I was 15 sheets to the wind by the time they started handing out awards. The first was for the best costume, which went to the PA to one of the executives; she was looking rather smouldering as a geisha, so no surprise there. I have an embarrassing recollection of proposing she and I have a quick wrestle, but unsurprisingly she turned me down. What was a surprise, however, was hearing my name over the PA system.

'Huh?' I asked the colleague who was standing closest to me, with all the eloquence I could muster given my blood alcohol level.

'Dude!' he said, swaying as if he were standing on the deck of an ocean liner in a storm. 'You won closer of the year! Great stuff.'

Through my alcohol-fuelled haze, it came back to me: I had, in fact, done a couple of shit-hot deals that year, and it did stand to reason that I would be recognised for some of the money I had earned for the company. I stumbled my way to the stage, and gratefully received an Xbox 360 (they had only just been launched, if I recall correctly) for my efforts.

Ace. A load of free booze and an Xbox 360, too? Tonight was turning out to be a much better evening than expected.

A few hours later, my friends decided that I had consumed quite enough alcohol for the rest of the year, and shoved me out the front door in the general direction of a row of waiting taxis. I don't recall putting up too much of a struggle, which probably was an indication that I had, indeed, had enough to drink for an evening.

I didn't live far away from the venue, so I decided to walk home instead of taking the cab. With my coat under one arm and my brand-new Xbox 360 under the other, I took off into the freezing cold December night in my slightly red-wine-stained judo gi.

I nearly made it home.

Nearly.

Suddenly, out of nowhere, a guy dressed like a ninja appeared. He was dressed all in black, with a raised hood. All I could see was his eyes as he squared up to me.

'Oi. Are you some sort of karate champion, then?' he said.

In retrospect, I should have seen that for what it was: a threat.

Instead, I started a profoundly incoherent tirade in which I intended to compare and contrast the differences between karate and judo. I believe I may have got as far as six syllables into my diatribe, when he took a step forward, and clocked me square in the face.

I woke up a couple of minutes later.

Blood was pouring from my nose, my Xbox 360 was gone, and I was resting against a brick wall, my coat over me for warmth.

'An ambulance is on the way,' a female voice said. I looked up at her.

She was cute.

I asked for her phone number, and she sighed, ignoring me. I told her to cancel the ambulance, but as I did so, I heard a siren coming closer. It was a police car.

'What happened to you?' the constable asked.

'I was attacked by a ninja,' I said, fully in earnest. The constable looked at me.

'Riiiight. How about you come and tell us about it at the station tomorrow. You look like you could do with some sleep.' The constable asked where I lived and I told him.

'That's only up the road,' he said, pointing at my house.

'Yeah, I know,' I said, adding drily: 'I live there.'

The next morning, I went to the police station to report being mugged for my games console . . .

The main reason I'm telling you this story is to illustrate the kind of things we sometimes have reported to us; people come in to the front office with all sorts of grievances, spanning from the most inane, inconsequential complaints to the most serious of crimes.

It's extremely hard to keep a straight face sometimes, and I'll admit that if someone had walked into my police station and told me that they had been attacked by a ninja, I would probably have sighed rather deeply myself. 'Not another one . . .'

I'll be honest. I'm not proud of this episode; I acted like a prat, drank far too much, and should have been more street-wise than walking home alone through a dodgy part of town with an expensive, shiny piece of kit under my arm.

The moral of the story is that not everybody who sounds like a complete nutjob is.

Only most of 'em.

The mysterious case of the Belgian bike burglar

'Two-six receiving Mike Delta,' my radio buzzed. I was slumped in the driver's seat of my Astra, which I'd parked in an employees-only car park behind a local shopping centre. Kim was snoozing in the seat next to me.

We were coming to the end of a 12-hour shift and bloody knackered. It was one of the last shifts on an unusually difficult pattern. All the officers were running at about 60 per cent mental capacity, which makes policing particularly difficult, because in many of the situations we run into we've really got to have our wits about us.

'Two-six. Two-six. Are you receiving, Mike Delta?' the radio buzzed again.

'Shit, that's us,' I realised, shaking my head. Had I been sleeping? I looked down at my hand; my coffee cup was precariously balanced on my lap, nearly – but not quite – tipping its scalding hot contents onto my leg. I straightened the cup carefully, and reached for the PTT lever on the dash.

'Yeah, two-six receiving. I apologise for the delay,' I added, 'I was on a private call.'

I immediately regretted lying to the CAD operator. They, and anybody else who had overheard that conversation, would have known it was a lie – we never apologise for delays in getting back to the CAD operator; either you respond in good time, or you're too busy to respond (for example, if you're in the middle of an arrest) and you'll call up as soon as you can.

'Er, yeah. Right. We've had a call about a theft. Shoplifter. You guys free?'

'At your service!' I said as brightly as I could. Next to me, Kim stretched and yawned, before zipping up her Metvest and fastening her seatbelt.

'Great, on its way to your MDT,' the operator said, just before the Mobile Data Terminal in our car used its ghastly pre-recorded voice to announce that the CAD had been updated.

Kim pressed the touch-screen on the MDT.

'The Bike Shack in Main Street detained a shoplifter, apparently, but then he got away,' she said.

'Call the bike shop, get a description,' I replied. We weren't that far away from Main Street, so I flicked the blue lights on and placed my coffee in the car's cup holder.

Kim made the call on speakerphone, so she wouldn't have to relay the description to me later. Clever.

'He was wearing a bright red T-shirt,' I heard Kim's radio say. 'And stole a very distinctive bike. It's a large-tubed bike, and the owner had taken all the paint off, sand-blasting the tubes to bare aluminium.'

As the bike shop manager continued his description, we went through a red light, sirens blaring. Suddenly, Kim made a squeaking sound – she does that when she can't think of words to describe what's going on – and pointed at the intersection we had just gone through. I slammed on the brakes, and looked in the direction of her gesticulations. There he was. Bright red T-shirt with a white logo on the front, and a bike that gleamed in the bright August sun. He had calmly stopped, letting us fly through the intersection unimpeded.

'I'll call you back,' Kim blurted at the bike shop owner, cancelling the call and getting straight back on the radio.

'Mike Delta receiving two-six,' she said.

'Go ahead.'

'We see a possible suspect for our bike theft; he's crossing Main Street at City Road, going east. We're just spinning the car around now. He's wearing a red tee, and riding an aluminium-coloured bike,' she said.

'Any units in the area who can assist with the last?' the operator asked.

'Show six-eight,' responded a gruff voice I recognised as Simon. 'One minute.'

Six-eight is the caged van we use for transporting prisoners. Excellent.

I could hear Simon's sirens come on at the far side of City Road, just as I had managed to turn my Astra around. I half expected a bit of a chase, but the cyclist simply stopped, pulling his bike half up on the pavement to let us pass him. He seemed a little bit confused when we came to a stop next to him.

Kim leapt out of the car and took a firm grip of his bike, before asking the suspect to please wait there. Simon arrived not ten seconds later, and stepped out of the van, along with his operator.

'Do you know why we've stopped you?' Kim asked.

'I suspect it is because of my bike,' he said.

'That's correct,' Kim said. 'Do you know why, specifically?'

'I'm guessing because I just took it from the bike shop up the road,' he said.

'Did you have permission to take the bike? A test ride, perhaps?' Kim said.

Confessions of a Police Constable

'No,' he said, and I saw Kim start reaching for her handcuffs. 'It's my bike, though. It was stolen from me.'

'Riiii-*ight*,' Kim said. 'Well, we are going to need to figure out exactly what has happened. I'm arresting you for theft; the arrest is necessary in order to assure a prompt and effective investigation. You do not have to say anything, but it may harm your defence if you don't mention, when questioned, something which you later rely on in court. Anything you do say may be given in evidence.'

'Yeah, yeah. But I can explain—' the man began.

'Time of arrest is eleven forty-six,' Kim interrupted, writing the time on the back of her hand with her biro.

Simon tapped my shoulder and beckoned me to step aside for a second.

'Cells are full, mate. We just had to take someone to Yankee Romeo, and that was the last of their cells, as well. We'll be taking bodies[25] to Essex next,' he huffed.

Yankee Romeo is the borough code for Lewisham – and it's nowhere near our own borough. It was no big surprise that cells were full everywhere: many boroughs had been doing a series of raids at the homes of people identified, thanks to CCTV, as having been involved in recent riots across London. However, having to take our prisoner all the way outside the Metropolitan Police area because of full cells would be a royal pain, not least because there was only 15 minutes left of my shift, and a trip to Essex would mean several hours' overtime. Usually, I'd welcome the overtime for the wage bump it implies, but after my tenth straight 12-hour shift, I'd gladly have paid to be able to go home and sleep for a few . . . well . . . *days*.

---

[25] 'Bodies' is police slang for prisoners; not, as some people assume, people headed for the morgue.

'I don't really fancy a two-hour round-trip,' I said. Simon grunted in agreement.

'Kim,' I said, 'can you put the guy in the cage for now? I'm going to try and find out what we need to do with him.'

Kim lead our prisoner to the van's back doors, as Simon took the bike and put it in the middle section. I reached for my radio.

'Is there a duty skipper available?' I asked.

'Unit calling for duty skipper,' replied the CAD operator. 'Please call up Mike Delta eight-eight.'

'Received,' I transmitted. 'Eight-eight receiving five-nine-two'.

'Eight-eight receiving, go ahead.'

'Spare please.'

'Changing,' the sergeant replied. I changed my radio to the spare channel.

'Mike Delta five-nine-two receiving.'

'Hi skip, I'm here. We've just arrested a suspected bike thief, but he claims the bike is his.'

'Yeah?'

'Well, I was just wondering if it would be okay to take him to the bike shop and see if we can square things up there; I don't really fancy a trip to Essex.'

'The clock's running, Matt,' the sergeant said, his voice garbled with exhaustion.

Someone later told me that this particular sergeant had recently finished an 18-hour shift, had six hours' sleep, and gone straight in for another 14 hours. Some of the skippers were completely unstoppable; bloody superheroes, the lot of them. The clock he was referring to is the force target of getting prisoners to custody within an hour of arrest.

'But yeah, knock yourself out,' he added. 'Keep me posted.'

'Thanks, sarge,' I said.

'Out,' he replied, and vanished from the spare channel.

I walked to the back of the police van.

'What's your name, mate?' I said.

'It's Case Jacobs,' he said.

'Case?' I replied. 'Unusual name, where's that from?'

'It's spelled K-E-E-S,' he said. 'I'm from Belgium.'

'Nice to meet you, Kees,' I said. 'Normally, we'd have taken you straight to a police station, but I propose we go talk to the bicycle shop owner first. Is that okay by you?'

'Of course,' he said.

'Good,' I said, closing the back doors on the caged Transit van, before throwing the keys to the Astra to Kim and climbing into the van through the side door.

Simon and Kim drove the vehicles to the bike shop, whilst I had a quick chat with Kees in the back of the Transit van.

'So, what happened, then?'

'I went into the bike shop to buy a new lock, as my last one was cut in half by the thieves, and I saw my bike there! I told the shop owner, but he said it wasn't my bike and that I couldn't have it back. So I took it.'

'How can you know it's your bike?' I asked.

'Look at it!' he laughed. 'Have you ever seen a bike like that? I fixed it up myself. There's no way that's not my bike. I changed the seat, and I can tell you every detail of every part of that bike.'

Then began a monologue about the various bits and pieces he had used to make it 'the perfect bike'.

'It has Shimano XTR components all around, even the chain,' he said, 'but I blasted off the markings so thieves wouldn't see them,' he said.

I took a closer look at the bike; true enough, every part was gleaming from having been sandblasted, and no markings were visible anywhere.

'That puts us in a bit of a weird situation, though,' I said. 'You say you've done it so thieves won't know that the bike is valuable, right?'

Kees replied with a nod.

'But that's a pretty common thing for thieves to do as well, so owners won't recognise their own bikes . . .'

We arrived at the bike shop.

'Hang on here for a second,' I told Kees. 'I'm just going to have a chat with the owner.' I turned to Kim, who'd just finished calling in an update about our situation. 'Wanna keep our friend company?' I asked.

'Yeah, sure,' she said, and walked to the back of the van, opening one of the doors to give our prisoner some fresh air.

I walked into the bike shop. The owner was there, looking none too pleased.

'Took you fucking long enough,' he said.

'True,' I said. 'But we caught the guy.'

The shopkeeper did a double take, then leaned forward and looked at the van. He couldn't see into it.

'Seriously?'

'Yeah, we spotted him as he was cycling along, so we stopped him.'

'Wow, that's great!'

'One little thing, though: he says the bike is his.'

'Yeah, he told me the same,' the shopkeeper said. 'But no . . . no way. Some kid brought it in the other day to get a flat tyre fixed.'

'In your opinion,' I said, 'is that a valuable bike?'

'It's a funny one, actually,' the shopkeeper said. 'It's a pretty standard Cannondale. They're popular bikes, but it's a mid-range bike, not usually particularly expensive. This particular one has had just about every component upgraded, though – high-end everything.'

'Did you do the upgrades for him?' I asked.

'Nope,' he replied. 'I've never seen the bike before.'

'Is it hard to replace a flat tyre?' I asked.

'No! Not at all.'

'It seems to me that this bike would have been owned by a bike lover, wouldn't you say?'

'Yeah, definitely. It came in super-clean. Seems as if the kid really loved his bike, definitely kept it in pristine condition.'

'So, forgive me if I'm asking a silly question – if someone is a huge bike fan, wouldn't they just replace their own inner tubes?' I asked.

'Yeah, I suppose so. But people are weird, y'know,' he shrugged.

'I don't suppose you have CCTV, do you?'

'Are you joking? We're CCTV'd to the rafters. I've got several bikes in here that are worth thousands and thousands of pounds; no way would I not have CCTV,' he said. 'In fact, I already took a look at the footage of the guy who brought the bike in, and of the fellow who nicked it.'

'Can I have a look?' I asked.

'Sure,' he replied, and waved me to the back of the shop.

It took me all of six seconds of the first video to recognise the lad who had brought the bike in for repair.

'I've got some bad news for you,' I said. 'That's Tommy, he's a drug addict and a notorious bike thief around here.'

'Seriously?' the owner said. 'I've seen him around the shop several times. He's never stolen anything,' he added, before pausing for several seconds. 'I don't think . . .'

'It doesn't mean anything,' I added. 'I haven't heard of him getting nicked for a good while, perhaps he's taken the straight and narrow . . .'

The shop owner shrugged and queued up the next video.

'Here you go,' he said. 'The guy had a funny accent. German

or something. He came in to buy a lock, but then he spotted the bike . . .'

The video didn't have sound, but it was unusually clear for CCTV. Surprisingly so, in fact. A lot of the CCTV footage we see is utterly useless, and some of it looks like it has been scrambled to hell and back, as if the entire file has been run through the blocking-out filter they apply to genitalia in Japanese pornography. Not that I would know what that looks like, of course.

In the video, I could clearly see Kees getting more and more aggravated. At one point, he simply takes the bike out of the rack, rips off a label that was zip-tied to the seat and starts pushing the bike towards the doors. The shop owner quickly blocks his way, but Kees runs his bike into the owner, before taking a swing at him with the lock he is holding in his hand.

'Stop there for a moment,' I said, and took a closer look at the shopkeeper. 'Did he hit you with the lock?' I asked him, looking at his face carefully.

'Yeah. He didn't hit me properly, though. That would have hurt,' he replied, as he lifted his hand to his face, rubbing his chin.

'Your eye still looks a bit swollen,' I said, thoughtfully.

'Yeah, well, I've had worse,' the shopkeeper said grimly. I looked at him, waiting for the rest of the story.

'Rugby,' he said, and grinned.

I smiled back.

'Hah, yeah, that makes sense,' I said. 'Would you excuse me for a moment?'

I went back to the van.

'Kees, do you have any receipts or anything for the bike?' I asked.

'Do you have an iPhone?' he replied.

'What for?' I asked, confused.

'I love my bike,' he replied, 'and I've kept a blog of all the work

I've done on it. The website I keep for my bike has all the receipts on it as well,' he said.

'Well, damn . . .' I said.

'I've run the bike through the box,' Kim said. 'It was reported stolen six days ago, by Kees here, and the serial number of the bike matches up with the police report. Also, when he filed his report, he showed the original purchase receipt of the bike, which matched the serial number as well.'

'Oh,' said Kees, 'and if you still doubt it, take the seat stem out of the bike'.

I walked around to the bike, unlocked the quick-release clasp, and took the seat off the bike. It looked pretty normal to me.

'What am I looking for here?' I asked.

'Look inside,' Kees said.

I felt around the bottom of the seat stem with my finger, and found something. I took it out and took a look. It was a piece of laminated paper that read: 'Property of Kees Jacobs', with a telephone number.

'It's a normal thing to do in Belgium,' Kees said, with a shrug.

'Hang on a sec,' I said, and went back to the bike shop.

'I'm starting to believe that the bike belongs to the "thief",' I told the shopkeeper. 'He reported it stolen six days ago. When did the lad drop it off to have the tyre fixed?'

The shopkeeper picked up the piece of paper that Kees had torn off the bike, and read it.

'Six days ago,' he said.

'So it seems as if someone stole the bike whilst the riots were raging, and Tommy dropped it off at your shop to get the tyre fixed soon after,' I said.

'Well . . . Fuck,' the proprietor contributed, summarising the culmination of our predicament perfectly.

'Yeah,' I agreed.

'We'll take the bike to the station, as it's stolen property. The owner can come and claim it when they produce their receipt,' I said.

'I bloody hate bike thieves,' he said.

'Yeah, I imagine you must do,' I replied. I paused, and looked at the shopkeeper for a few moments. His eye had swollen even further. The words 'Crikey, that's gonna hurt in the mornin', son' from that annoying Fosters advert echoed around in my head.

'That leaves only one thing,' I said. 'The bike owner assaulted you. We have all the evidence we need to prosecute him, I think. All we need is your video footage, and a statement . . .'

'Ah,' the shopkeeper said, rubbing the side of his head. 'You're positive he's not a bike thief?'

'You can never be sure,' I said. 'But he does seem to have all the receipts to back up his claims. He bought most of the parts off eBay and put the whole bike together himself. He showed me a blog of the work in progress; it looks like it all checks out.'

'Can I talk to him?' he asked.

I hesitated.

'Not really, to be honest. If we're going to charge him, we need to interview him at the police station.'

'Can I go stand by your van and just think out loud for a bit, then?' he asked, with a conspiratory smile on his face.

'Do you have a bathroom?' I asked.

'I do,' he said, pointing with his thumb towards a door in the corner of his workshop.

'I'm going to go use the loo, then, if you don't mind. What you do whilst I'm gone is up to you, really,' I said, and walked to the bathroom.

When I came back out, the shopkeeper was standing next to the van, laughing with Kim.

Kim came up to me.

'The shopkeeper is refusing to make a statement about the

assault, and says that he may have "accidentally" deleted the footage of it,' she said. 'What should we do?'

'Well, if there's no evidence of an assault, no allegations of any sort . . .' I said, adding: 'Obviously, Kees can't have stolen his own bike.'

Kim let our suspect out of the caged van but kept him in handcuffs.

'So, just to confirm, I've written here: "I, Dan Smith, proprietor of the Bike Shack on seventy-three Main Street, confirm that I do not allege any crimes in connection with my 999 call. CAD eight-seven-four-nine refers". If that sounds accurate, all you need to do is to sign here, and we'll be out of your hair,' I said.

'Yeah, no worries. Turns out Kees and I have friends in common, and to be honest, I'd punch anyone who got in the way of stealing my pride and joy as well,' he said, laughing.

'Just for future reference,' I said, 'I probably wouldn't say that to a police officer if I were you. What he should have done is to dial 999 himself; that would have solved the whole incident without anyone getting any black eyes.'

'Yeah, of course. Of course,' the shopkeeper said, as he signed and dated my pocketbook. 'Keep up the good work, officer!' he added, and walked off.

'Get some ice on that eye,' I called after him. He raised a hand and waved a thank you, as he strolled back to his shop. I doubted he would actually bother with the ice.

'Kees,' I said, turning to the young man, who was leant against the police van, flirting with Kim.

'Yes, sir?'

'We've got a bit of a problem,' I said. 'The shopkeeper showed me some CCTV footage of what happened in the shop. You took a swing at him with a bike lock and hit him across the face.'

Kees nodded gravely.

'That's assault. Given the bruising on his face, I'm guessing you could be charged with ABH – actual bodily harm. That's pretty serious stuff,' I said, keeping my eyes locked in his. 'Serious enough, in fact, that if you were convicted, you could face several years in prison.'

Kees went notably paler as I was talking to him, and started stuttering an apology.

'Please just listen to me. In this case, the correct thing to do would have been to call the police, and tell them that you had found your bike. We would have been there in a flash, and we'd have gotten your bike back. See it from the shopkeeper's side: he was protecting the property that he thought belonged to a customer. From his perspective – no matter what you said to him – you were trying to steal that bike. Instead of solving this like an adult, because of the choices you made, you ended up hitting a man who hates bike thieves as much as you do. You're very lucky that he is refusing to make a statement. Things could have been very different; that D-lock is heavy, and you could have easily broken his jaw, or even killed him if you had been even less lucky. Or he might have given a statement and given us the CCTV. And there's no way you could have claimed self-defence or anything like that either, because it was your fault that the situation escalated.'

As the gravity of the situation dawned on Kees, he got more and more pale. I opened the door of the police van and asked if he would like to sit down on the step. He accepted.

'I'm going to do a "street bail", which means I'm going to let you go, but you'll need to show up at the police station so we can give you a formal warning,' I said and explained to him how much trouble he would be in if he missed his appointment, and that he would have to come to the police station to pick up his bike anyway.

'Come to the station the day after tomorrow at three. We'll sort out your caution. That's going to go on your police record, by the way, but it's not a criminal conviction. I'll explain all of that to you when you come to the station,' I said. 'Bring the receipts for your bike as well, and we'll make sure you get your bike back. Do you have any questions?' I finished.

He shook his pale face slowly.

'Right, let's get these cuffs off you, then,' I said, and freed him, before passing Kim's cuffs back to her.

'Off you go, and see you the day after tomorrow,' I said. Kees nodded, but seemed to be in a complete daze.

'First time you've talked to the police?' Kim asked him. He nodded.

'Well, second, actually,' he said. 'The first time was last week, when I reported my bike stolen.'

'Don't worry too much about it,' she said. 'Assault is serious, but I'm guessing you've learned your lesson, right?'

Kees nodded vigorously.

'You'll get a warning out of it, but it could have been much, much worse. Just remember for the next time, that violence probably isn't going to solve anything, all right?'

Kees nodded again.

'Thank you,' he said to Kim, before turning to me. 'Thank you,' he repeated.

'No worries. See you the day after tomorrow,' I said. 'And stay out of trouble, all right?'

'Yes, sir!' he said.

To my confusion, he did a military-style salute to both of us, before he walked off, dialling a number on his phone.

Is that a baton you have in your pocket?

One of the most common questions from civilians is: 'What do you carry around with you when you're on duty?'

The simplest answer is: 'Lots!'

I carry general first aid stuff, a lot of gloves, my Police Pocketbook, a stack of Fixed Penalty Notices, my Collision and Accident Report Book, Evidence and Action Book, stop-and-search forms, domestic violence process books, and about half a dozen other pieces of paper, forms and booklets.

In addition to being three-quarters of a walking filing cabinet, I carry plenty of gadgets with me; unsurprisingly, it appears that people tend to find the technological baggage more interesting than the half-tonne of dead trees.

My Personal Protection Kit consists of:

My Metvest – A slash and ballistic vest that is designed to protect us against slashing and stabbing attacks and small-calibre gunfire. It's also good as general impact protection; one of my colleagues once received the business end of a cricket bat across her back, and she walked away from it. Without the Metvest, she would, at the very least, have spent a long night in A&E. But as far as I can tell, the Metvest's primary purpose is to make you sweat like a randy otter, and provide some nice big pockets you can use to carry the 600 forms you need on an average shift.

The ASP – Back in the mists of time, the Met only used one brand of baton, made by a company called Armament Systems and Procedures. These batons had ASP written on the side of them. Today, even though the current-issue batons are made by a completely different company called Monadnock, everybody still refers to them as Asps. My baton is a 21-inch telescopic friction-lock extendable baton – or a GFLB (the G in GFLB refers to 'gravity' – as opposed to spring-loaded friction-lock batons – and the FLB is a Friction-Lock Baton).

It's a clever piece of kit; it stays out of the way most of the time, but when you need it, it's reassuring to have 21 inches of steel at your beck and call.

When it comes to the batons, every six months we do a fair bit of training with them, as part of our OST[26]. I'm glad to report that, whilst I won't hesitate to 'rack' my baton if the situation calls for it, I haven't had to use it all that often.

CS Spray – In addition to the Asp, we're issued with a small canister of CS[27] spray. Under English law, it is technically defined as a firearm, as is 'any weapon designed for the discharge of any noxious liquid'. Our canisters don't fire the thin mist you'd expect from, say, a spray deodorant; instead, they project a stream of liquid, much like a water pistol. CS is a curious weapon to issue us with: roughly ten per cent of the population have very little response to

---

[26] Officer Safety Training

[27] CS is technically o-chlorobenzylidene malononitrile – but the letters C and S refer to Corson and Stoughton, the two Americans who discovered the compound.

CS gas. At the other end of the scale, ten per cent react extremely to it.

In training, we all have to 'get gassed' ourselves, so that we understand what the effects are, how long they last, and what you have to do to make it wear off as quickly as possible. It turns out that my reaction to CS is at the extreme end of the scale, a situation that is not helped by the fact that I wear contact lenses when I'm on duty. Whenever CS is used on duty, everyone on scene is likely to be subjected to at least a little bit of the stuff as well, and when I am, I'm on the floor with tears, snot and sweat flowing everywhere. Not very dignified, and perhaps the main reason I have never discharged my own CS – I know that for me it is a rubbish tactical option.

Handcuffs – Finally, I've got a set of lovely Hiatt Speedcuffs. As I explained earlier, these are rigid handcuffs (as opposed to the ones with a chain between each wrist), and they're rather nifty. They're quite clunky to carry around with you, but they are solid enough to be used as a weapon if required. If I'm approaching a suspect holding a set of handcuffs and they suddenly turn violent, it's more economical, time-wise, to give them a couple of jabs with my cuffs than to have to take a step back, put my cuffs away and reach for my baton.

I'd say that my handcuffs are probably my most oft-used piece of PPE[28]; I use them several times per week, whereas I might draw my baton only a few times per month, and my CS has stayed in its holster for as long as I've had it.

It stands to reason that, since I carry a good 15 kilos of paperwork and other crap with me, it's pretty hard to run in all

[28] Personal Protection Equipment

this equipment. Even the fastest, fittest of police officers will not stand a chance against a 17-year-old in his physical prime weighed down by only a tracksuit and a pair of running shoes. And, it saddens me to say, I'm neither the fastest nor the fittest police officer on the Metropolitan Police payroll . . .

Not long ago, I was on holiday in the United States. I ended up in Chicago, in a rather, well, 'authentic' café. In the corner, there was a table of city officers, fresh from a shift.

I've always been a little curious about how real-life policing happens in the colonies. Feeling bold, I asked the gentlemen if I could join them for a bit.

'Uhm . . .yeah,' one of them said, uncertainly. I could see in his eyes he was considering telling me to *eff off* in a manner becoming of a Man in Blue, Chicago-style.

'It's okay, I'm a cop back in London,' I said. They seemed relieved, asked me to join them, bought me a beer and we got down to the business of comparing notes.

They got the ball rolling by telling me a little about the computer systems they use in the police cruisers. Suffice to say, they use laptops that are a damn sight more advanced than the stuff we have. These cops are able to do full-on police reports right there in the car, without having to go back to the station. Of course, our MDT[29] computers are useful, but they're not exactly fast to use; they are mostly just used by the CAD[30] dispatchers, plus the odd PNC[31] check.

So whilst these guys can finish up their paperwork on scene, at the end of a long day, I'm stuck waiting for a free computer in the writing room. There are eight computers, but five of them will

---

[29] Mobile Data Terminal
[30] Computer Aided Dispatch
[31] Police National Computer

invariably be out of service and the rest are old. The writing room also frequently reeks of weed – not because the coppers smoke it, but because people find it hilarious to bring the weed into the writing room in evidence bags to show off their haul, letting the smell seep into the pores of all their colleagues. All good and well, except that sniffer dogs at tube stations keep singling us out. It's just our sense of humour, I suppose.

Once I'd finished my grilling of the American officers, it was their turn to ask me a few questions. After confirming I worked in London, the first question was: 'So . . . when was the last time you shot anyone?'

I won't lie to you. I was completely stunned by the question. I have never been an authorised firearms officer (AFO) – in fact, I've scarcely even touched a handgun, never mind *fired* one, and I've certainly not shot one *at* somebody.

I must have given away my confusion pretty quickly: I think I may have been opening and closing my mouth like a fish on dry land, because the US coppers burst out laughing.

'Well . . .' I countered. 'Have you *all* shot someone?'

'I haven't,' one of the younger cops said, with a look of regret on his 20-year-old face.

'But I'm the only one,' he added, with an embarrassed glance around the rest of the table.

What followed was a game of one-upmanship with tales about gun-drawn bravado in the line of duty. It was a very informative, interesting and entertaining afternoon. I explained to the Chicago officers the kind of kit I usually carry around on a day-to-day basis.

'So, you have a stick, a set of fashion faux-pas bangles and some particularly nasty deodorant, basically?' one of them had asked.

In short: yes. Still, I'll be the first to admit that I'm rather glad

I am never faced with the choice of whether or not I need to shoot a suspect.

I do have one more 'weapon', however, which comes in handy every now and again: my radio. It has a red button on it that I can press when it all goes a bit Pete Tong; for example, if I'm facing a psycho with a pistol, a nutter with a knife, or a madman with a machete (it *has* happened). A quick press of that button and a shout for Trojan (armed police) assistance, and the guys with the guns come flying in their BMW 5-shaped ARVs[32].

The radios we use are Motorola MTH800 units, operating on the Airwave network. They're generally pretty good, apart from the fact that they don't work very well indoors. They are particularly useless in some of the lovely council-provided habitation facilities on my borough. Pretty unfortunate considering this is precisely where things have a tendency to go wrong.

As far as weaponry goes, I know that a lot of coppers are in favour of us being armed with Tasers, or even that more constables should be routinely armed with firearms. Personally, I don't really see the point. If all police start carrying weapons, I imagine the criminals we are up against are going to escalate their side of the arms race as well. As it is, I don't think I've been in many situations where it would have been helpful for me to carry an oversized bug-zapper with me.

[32] Armed Response Vehicle

Tinker, Tailor . . . Spy?

In this job, every once in a while you come across cases that are just plain bizarre. There was the 12-year-old I arrested for sexual assault, the 80-year-old that got nicked for stealing fully-inflated party balloons (he'd tried to do a runner with his Zimmer frame), and the car thief I completely failed to arrest because she flashed her boobs: she caused such a stir amongst a group of bystanders that I was distracted for long enough for her to simply leave the car where it was, saunter off and get on the tube.

From the moment I spotted Jamie, I knew there was something just a little bit odd about him. I just wasn't able to pinpoint what. He drove meticulously, with both his hands on the steering wheel, and he seemed to drive to 'the system', much like they teach us in our advanced driving course. And then there was his demeanour when I pulled him over for talking on his mobile phone whilst driving . . .

It all started after I had just finished taking a burglary statement. Usually, it would be the Burglary Squad who dealt with burglaries, unsurprisingly (I'll leave it to your imagination what the Licensing Division or the Robbery Taskforce do . . .). However, this particular theft victim had been so desperately upset, the operator had upgraded our response and sent me over to take an initial statement. It was a relatively QT[33] shift, and the Burglary team were swamped thanks to a spate of non-residential burglaries on the borough.

As I was pulling back onto the main road, I spotted somebody doing something they shouldn't be doing whilst driving, and since I was officially 'on patrol', I figured I'd pull them over and have a chat.

'Please turn off your ignition, leave your keys in the car and join me on the pavement,' I asked the driver, after walking up to his passenger-side window. He shrugged, killed the engine on his car, took his keys out of the ignition, looked carefully to see if there were any cars coming, then got out, walked around and leaned against the slightly battered but overall well-maintained Audi A4 saloon.

'Do you know why I stopped you?' I asked him, in that fishing-for-self-incriminatory-information kind of way that I seemed to perfect the day I graduated from Hendon.

'I believe I do,' he said, to my surprise. 'I was talking on my mobile phone, contravening section 26 of the Road Safety Act of 2006 and, I suppose, regulation 104 of the Road Vehicles Regulations of 1986, officer.' He flashed a half-smile at me, which I wasn't quite able to ascertain the meaning of.

Surprisingly, it isn't often I stare into the face of a man who knows exactly what he has been stopped for down to the act and regulation. Usually, people pretend to not have spoken on the phone (a daft move, it's pretty easy to see when you're driving behind somebody). When that defence fails, they pretend they didn't know it was illegal, and when *that* doesn't work, they usually

---

[33] Saying the Q-word to mean 'the opposite of busy' is bad luck in this job; whenever someone exclaims, 'My, is it quiet today', it invariably means that the rest of the shift descends into a shitstorm of historical proportions. The last time someone mentioned the Q-word over the radio, the riots broke out a few hours later. QT stands for Quiet Time.

tell me that they've never done it before, that it was a really important call, and that they will never do it again if they please, please, please don't get a ticket because their insurance is going to go up if I issue one.

It's not that I'm not sympathetic to these things. Over the years, the Black Rats[34] have caught me for a small yet illustrious menu of motoring offences, including speeding and being on the car phone whilst driving (car phones! Does anyone even remember those?). After I started this job, I put a swift end to silliness behind the wheel. Part of what I do for a living is attend traffic collisions, and it is easily my least favourite part of the job – and, indeed, of my life as a whole.

The truth is, traffic 'accidents' are caused by technical failure only in extremely rare cases. The two biggest reasons for accidents in traffic are stupidity and complacence. The combination of these two things is a particularly nasty cocktail. Just because you've driven yourself to work every day for the past three years without an incident, it doesn't mean that a cyclist isn't going to be on your left as you turn without looking. It doesn't mean that you can text your friend about your plans for the weekend because there wasn't a kid playing in that particular part of the road the day before. It doesn't mean you can put in your contact lenses whilst driving because you didn't have time before you jumped in the car. I've seen all three of these things happen.

Normally after I ask someone whether they know why I stopped them, I explain all these things to them: nobody likes being stopped by the police, nobody likes to get a ticket, and I understand it when people get grumpy about being caught out. Nonetheless, I won't apologise – endanger my roads where I can see you, and you're fair game.

But I digress.

[34] Traffic police

Jamie was standing there, hands in his jeans pockets, as my radio buzzed into life.

'Five-nine-two receiving Mike Delta,' it chimed. I turned the volume down a couple of clicks before responding.

'Five-nine-two receiving.'

'Are you still on scene?'

'Yes, yes. I'll be about twenty minutes.'

'Are you Charlie Papa?'

Now, I should explain that the last question normally means trouble. Charlie Papa is short for Close Proximity, which means that they want to talk to me without my suspect overhearing it. This usually means that they've found a marker on the person or the car that I am dealing with, and have a piece of news that I need to know about. I've already run his plates through the system, so the operator will know all about the vehicle and its owner. They may need to tell me that there is a warrant for his arrest, or that he is known for guns or violence.

'Spare, please,' I requested.

'Changing,' the CAD operator replied, and I change my radio to the spare channel.

'Jamie, I won't be a minute,' I said, and walked out of earshot.

'No worries, take your time,' he said, still leaning against the grey Audi, and now fiddling with, but not lighting, a cigarette.

'Can you repeat the index, please,' the CAD operator asked me. She wants me to read out the number plate again.

'Yes, yes. It's Kilo Alpha Five Four Mike Bravo X-Ray.'

'Stand by,' the CAD operator said before the radio went quiet. After what seems like an eternity, the operator came back on.

'Five-nine-two receiving,' she said.

'Go ahead,' I replied.

'Er, there's a marker on the car, do you have your mobile on you?' It's an unusual request; why would I need my mobile phone?

'Yes,' I replied, and hesitantly added '. . . Is everything okay?'

'Stand by your mobile,' was her only reply. 'Mike Delta out.'

The busy A-road was buzzing with traffic pulling past us at a slow pace. The park behind me sent a fresh breeze my way, and Jamie was finally lighting the cigarette he had been playing with, never taking his eyes off me for a second.

I switched my radio back to the main dispatch channel, and just as I finished doing that, my phone rang with a withheld number.

'Hi, is that Delito five-nine-two Mike Delta?'

'Umm . . . Yes, it is. Who is speaking, please?'

'Yeah, this is Commander Smith from CO fifteen.' My brain was racing. CO15 is the counter-terrorism unit: what the hell would they want from me, and why do I suddenly have a commander on the line?

'We just had a phone call from special branch. Did you just tug[35] Kilo Alpha Five Four Mike Bravo X-Ray?'

'Er . . . Yes, sir, I did.'

'Who is the driver of the vehicle?' I glanced over at Jamie. Is he a terrorist? What the hell is going on?

'It's a Jamie, sir . . .' I read the name on the licence. 'Cancel that. His name is James Robert McKenzie, sir.'

'Okay, that's all right,' the man on the phone said.

'Jamie is a good man. What did you stop him for?' he asked.

'He was driving whilst talking on his mobile, sir,' I replied.

'That's fine. Give him a ticket, but don't run his name through PNC. Once he's left, make sure to destroy the ticket, and please give me a call once you're back in the office.'

Commander Smith rang off after giving me an internal Metropolitan Police telephone number. I checked with Dispatch to make sure that I was to do what the Commander had just told

[35] 'Tug' – to pull a car over.

me, and then I walked over to Jamie. I calmly started writing him out a £60 endorsable fixed penalty notice. I explained to him that he had to pay within 28 days, and that he would get three points on his licence. Jamie was completely unfazed by any of it. He listened politely – carefully, even – but didn't say a word.

Once the process was completed, he spoke.

'Thanks, buddy. Stay safe.' He extended his hand to shake mine, but I curtly shook my head; I wouldn't usually shake someone's hand after handing them a ticket – it's a safety thing. He shrugged, flashed me another smile and then climbed back into his car.

The silver Audi slid off the sidewalk and back into traffic.

Before he faded into the sea of metal, I spotted Jamie waving a greeting of thanks to the driver that let him in, and I kicked myself. I should have said or done something cool! I should have at least shook his hand.

Or perhaps invited him for a pint.

Or borrowed a cigarette off him.

I don't even smoke.

I tried to call Commander Smith but was instead greeted by an inspector who said he'd meet me at the police station for a debriefing in person. It turned out that the system should have flagged up a warning message as soon as I ran the car through the PNC (Police National Computer). Normally, the message that would have shown was: 'Must not be stopped without Trojan assistance', but due to a glitch that didn't happen.

They never did tell me who Jamie was or what he did (or, indeed, if that was his real name), only that he was not 'job' (so, not working for the police) but did work for the government.

Out of all the traffic stops I've done, Jamie is probably the only spy I've ever seen . . . That I know of.

Crossing over to the other side

'Call an ambulance,' I shouted, as I ran across the road to the man on the asphalt. He was making a horrible gargling sound. In the three seconds it took me to cross the road, his white T-shirt had been soaked with claret.

I applied pressure to his throat to try and stop the bleeding, but it kept coming out with a surprising amount of force; I didn't seem to be able to even slow the bleeding.

The passer-by I had shouted at for an ambulance was fumbling with her mobile phone. She said something, but not loud enough for me to hear. 'What?!' I barked back.

'I don't know the number,' she blurted out, and burst into tears.

There wasn't time to stop and ponder about the sheer idiocy of that statement. Even though I was now covered in blood trying to save the man's life, an old joke forced its way to the forefront of my mind: 'Operator! What is the number for 911?!'

It had all begun barely a minute earlier. I was on my way to a late shift. We were parading at two, so I left the house at about noon. I treated myself to a full English breakfast and a couple of cups of nuclear-strength java, before walking to work.

I was at an intersection. Traffic was backed up, so a couple of my fellow pedestrians took the opportunity to cross between the cars. As long as the road is clear, there's no problem with this; there are no laws against jaywalking in the UK.

I considered crossing myself, but I looked further up the road, and through the front windshield of a bus, I saw a motorcycle moving up the far side of the line of traffic at a lofty pace.

'A bit risky,' I remember thinking. A fraction of a second later, someone brushed past me, and darted in front of the white Transit van that was stopped in front of us.

His timing could not have been worse. I opened my mouth to warn the pedestrian about the motorcyclist, but before as much as a syllable had shaped in my vocal cords, I was interrupted by a sickening sound. The motorcycle's mirror was the first point of impact against the pedestrian. The force against the right handlebar made the motorbike turn right, and it crashed into the back of the car that had stopped just in front of the van, sending the motorcyclist sailing through the air.

The pedestrian went down like a sack of spuds. As he did, he smashed his head against the side of the pavement. He must have sliced his throat open against something on the motorcycle – before I even managed to make it over to him, he had grasped at his throat and then blacked out.

I shouted at the shocked lady: '999! It's 999! Call them now!' Her mobile was still in her hands, her eyes flicking between the motorcyclist who'd gone flying clean over the car he hit, and the pedestrian whose life was leaking out of the gaping gash in his throat.

Another passer-by held a phone to my ear.

'999, what is your emergency?' the operator asked. I glanced up at the passer-by. He was only a kid, perhaps 16 years old. He looked pale. I mouthed 'Thank you' to him, before turning my attention to the phone.

'This is Matthew Delito, PC five-nine-two Mike Delta. I need an ambulance.' The operator connected me to another – the dispatch unit for the ambulance service, I presumed. Meanwhile I was still trying to stop the blood gushing out of the pedestrian's throat, and not having much luck. His lips were going blue, he was getting weaker, and now his bleeding was slowing down.

'I have two casualties – one male, around twenty-four years of age, not responding, laboured breathing. He has severe neck trauma, bleeding profusely. The other is a motorcyclist.'

I glanced over at the motorcyclist. He was moaning and moving around, which meant he was hurt, but at least he was breathing. If a man's breathing it means his heart is beating. If his heart is beating, well, that means he's already better off than the pedestrian I was dealing with.

'The motorcyclist is conscious and breathing, but he's got unknown injuries. He went flying. Broken bones at least. Oh, and get some police over here, it's a fucking mess,' I finished.

A woman showed up out of nowhere and took the phone – now dripping with blood – from me. She asked if I was okay.

'Yeah, fine,' I barked, glancing desperately at the pedestrian who had stopped any attempts at breathing. She checked his pulse, and relayed something to the 999 operator who was still on the line.

'Could you go deal with the motorcyclist?' she asked me. 'I don't think there's a lot you can do here.' As she said this, she produced a pair of gloves out of her purse, put them on and took over from me, applying pressure to the man's throat.

I must have looked rather grateful, because she responded by smiling for a brief moment, before nodding her head towards the motorcyclist. 'Go save a life, cowboy,' she said.

I recognised her just as I made to turn away; we bring prisoners to A&E all the time and she was one of the nurses we deal with.

I shook my thoughts back to the task at hand as I bounded

over to the motorcyclist. His arm was sticking out at a curious angle. With his other, working, arm he was wrestling with his helmet.

'Hey. I'm police. Don't worry, an ambulance is on the way. I need you to lay down and not move for a while, okay?' He seemed happy to take instructions. 'What's your name, mate?' I asked him.

He said something that sounded like Alexej.

'Alex. Can I call you Alex?' He tried to nod, but I stopped him with a wave. 'Alex, you may have a neck injury, and nodding is bad news. I need you to lay down on your back and just not move. Can you do that for me?' He did. I opened up the visor of his helmet to give him some extra air. He was dazed but able to talk to me.

'The man. Is he okay?' Alex asked me, straining to move his head to catch a glimpse of the pedestrian.

'I don't know,' I lied, hoping Alex wouldn't notice that I looked like I'd been doing butterfly strokes in red paint all morning. 'The ambulance will deal with him. For now, I'm just worried about you. Where do you live, mate?' I talked to him about various day-to-day things, just to keep his mind occupied. Keeping him talking had an additional bonus: it meant that I would immediately notice if his situation worsened.

The first ambulance arrived, and I knew it was bad news when they came over to us nearly immediately.

'Let's have a look at you, then,' the paramedic said to the motorcyclist, before looking at me and shaking his head.

The pedestrian didn't make it.

It's always really hard not to place the blame in traffic collisions. In this case, the motorcyclist was going too fast for the conditions, but still well within the speed limit. As far as he was concerned, he was crossing on a green light, and making good progress past a line of stopped cars. The pedestrian only saw the line of stopped traffic, ignored the red light for pedestrians and failed to consider whether there might be other traffic behind the stopped vehicles. He should have stopped to check, perhaps, but it's easy to forget – even if it was an oversight that claimed his life that day.

More police and ambulances showed up; the motorcyclist had a badly broken arm and a serious concussion. I called my sergeant, and told him the state of play.

'Go home, Delito,' he said. 'We've got plenty of people on today, sounds like you need a break.'

I felt bad about leaving my team in the lurch; traffic accidents like this are relatively commonplace, and I could have worked my shift if I'd had to, but I was looking forward to a shower, to scrubbing the blood off me, to getting my clothes into a washing machine and going back to bed.

One of the ambulances gave me a lift home: it was on the way to the hospital anyway. I remember my last thought before I went to sleep was 'What a horrible way to die.'

'Going the Way of the Dojo'

In the parking lot behind a local Sainsbury's, I was sitting with my feet on the Panda's dashboard, waiting for my colleague Jay to come back with our lunch. I didn't really have any reason for staying in the car, other than complete, abject laziness. I suppose I quite like to have someone else buy my lunch for me . . . with my own money, of course.

Jay, especially, had been on a great streak for picking tasty foods lately – he'd had a vegan girlfriend for a while, a relationship that fell apart, and he'd been trying to take revenge by eating as many cows, lambs and chickens as possible. If you ask me, it's not the greatest way of getting back at an ex, but as long as it made him happy . . .

'Mike Delta two-four receiving Mike Delta,' the radio buzzed. I looked down lazily, before reaching for the in-car handset. It was one of those old-fashioned squeeze-button microphones you see in American cop shows a lot. We never use it; in fact, I'm not even sure why we have them. The cars are fitted with small microphones next to the sun visors, along with fancy push-to-talk buttons on the steering wheel – but I guess I was in a retro mood.

'Ten-four, Mike Delta,' I said, in my worst American accent. (Incidentally, that is also my best American accent.)

'You free to deal with an assault?'

'Yeah, why not. Send 'er over.'

'Done. Thanks. It's on an S-grade.'

'Received!'

I reached for my phone. The call was a Sierra-grade. This meant we had an hour to get to the location, but it never harms to get going. I rang Jay on his mobile, to urge him to get a move on. It's possible to call people directly radio-to-radio, of course, but the user interface on our radios is very Motorola circa 1995, which means it takes a rocket scientist to figure out how to programme numbers into the phone book etc. So I just went ahead and called him on my personal phone instead. At least that's usable.

Before long, Jay hopped into the car. From the second he opened the door, I was aware of a truly delicious smell.

'What'd you get?' I asked, fastening my seatbelt.

'Chicken. Roasted. Whole,' Jay replied. I looked over. He grinned, barely holding back from salivating. 'Where are we going, then?'

'Church Street,' I replied. 'It's a weird one, actually. We've been called to a boxing ring about an assault, I think. We're meeting a Chris there, who is the victim, apparently.'

We made it to the address we had been given in decent time.

'This,' Jay observed, 'is not a boxing gym.'

We were standing outside a deep and narrow building, with Japanese-looking writing on the signs and posters. This was a martial arts dojo, and a much fancier one than the ratty, 1960s-throwback community hall where I train jiu-jitsu twice per week.

A paramedic came out to greet us.

'This way,' he said, without seeming to be in a particular hurry. That's usually either really good news or really bad news: either Chris wasn't hurt enough to warrant being in a rush, or he had already died.

We were led into a café-looking area near the front of the dojo. An advanced session of some martial art I didn't recognise – it looked a little bit like taekwondo – was in progress in the hall itself. We could see the training through the large glass wall, and it looked rather impressive.

In the café, we met a young man in a martial arts costume. Another paramedic was checking his pulse and blood pressure, as he sat in a chair.

Not dead, then, I concluded.

'What happened here?' Jay asked, after we had introduced ourselves and verified that this was, indeed, Chris.

Chris opened his mouth to answer, and it was immediately clear that he had recently had a tooth knocked out, in addition to other injuries to his face – and arm, which he was wearing in a sling clutched close to his body.

'He beat the shit out of me,' Chris said.

'Who did?'

'The instructor.'

'What is his name?'

'John.'

'Where is he?'

'In there,' Chris nodded, starting to turn his head to look through the glass wall, but then flinching in pain as he twisted his neck.

'Right. So what exactly happened?'

'We were training, and I landed a punch a little bit too hard.'

'So you punched him?'

'Yeah, I suppose, but I didn't mean to. Or, well, I meant to punch him, just not as hard as I did.'

'Forgive me if I ask a stupid question,' Jay started, 'But isn't punching people the point of martial arts?'

'Well, yeah – but we don't go full contact without a lot of

padding. Normally, we just mark our punches, and I guess I miscalculated, and put a little bit too much into my punch.'

'By accident?'

'Of course!'

'Does that happen a lot?' Jay asked

'I suppose it's not uncommon to leave a session with a few bruises here and there. When you get better, you tend to have more control. As you climb through the belts you learn more, and you become used to not punching too hard. I guess I miscalculated in this case.'

'Right. And then what happened?'

'He paused for a second, pointed at me, and without saying anything, started beating me up.'

'And this is the instructor?'

'Yeah.'

'I see you're wearing a green belt.'

'With a blue stripe,' Chris replied, holding up the limp, blood-splattered end of his green belt, to show off a thin length of blue fabric that was attached.

'Whatever. What does that mean?'

'Er?'

'Does having a green belt with a blue stripe mean you know what you're doing?'

'I suppose it means I'm about halfway to my black belt,' Chris replied.

'And the instructor . . . he is a black belt?'

'Yeah. I don't know what dan, though.'

'Dan?' Jay turned to me: 'Matt, you know this stuff, don't you?'

'I dabble,' I said. 'Not in this sport, though.'

'Are injuries common?' Jay asked me.

'Not in jitsu.' I reply. 'Bruises, mostly.'

'Yeah, same here,' Chris said.

'So, he just went for you?' I asked Chris.

'Yeah. I hit him in the front of the shoulder. I suppose I may have hit his clavicle. He just lost his shit and went for me. I think he only got about six strikes in before the others dragged him off, but the doc here thinks he has broken my arm. He broke one of my teeth, too, and I'm definitely going to have a bit of a shiner as well. He kicked me in the head.'

'Did you fall down?' I asked.

'No, I was standing the whole time.'

'But he still kicked you in the head?'

Chris laughed. 'Kicking someone in the head when they're standing up isn't that hard,' he said.

In jitsu, we don't really bother with kicks above the belt level: if you're going to give up that much balance, you may as well get in close and break one of their joints. I suppose this is one of the philosophical differences between our two martial arts.

'And the instructor's name is John?' I checked.

'Yeah. He's the tall bald guy,' Chris said.

Jay and I stood at the window briefly, and watched the action on the other side of the glass.

'Let's do this,' he said, glancing over at me.

He unfastened the pushbutton that secures his CS gas and loosened his baton in his holster. I shook my head and did the same, before we both walked into the main arena.

'What is this?' John the instructor bellowed. 'Get those filthy shoes off our mats!'

I completely understood where he was coming from, and I felt genuinely guilty about tromping straight onto the mats. In martial arts, this is a place of respect: you bow to enter the dojo itself, then you bow again to walk out onto the mats, then you bow when you face an opponent – and you do it all again, in reverse, when you leave. In the context of most martial arts, wearing your shoes on the mats is quite spectacularly rude.

However, when we both hurriedly stepped back onto the solid ground, the instructor made no move to come join us.

'Can you come over here for a moment? We need to talk to you,' Jay said, resting his right hand on his handcuffs, beckoning for John to come closer.

'Can it wait?' John said, glancing at the clock mounted above the door we had just entered. 'We are finished in about forty minutes.'

''Fraid not,' Jay said. 'Now, please.'

'Seriously, forty minutes,' the instructor said, visibly annoyed.

'No.' Jay said. 'Now.'

The instructor still didn't appear to want to come over.

'Look, I really don't want to step on your mats again, but if I have to, I will. I need to talk to you, and we're going to do it like civilised people, not with five metres between us and fifteen people looking on.'

'They all saw what happened; they'll back me up,' John replied.

'My friend,' Jay started, 'you have ten seconds. I'm going to go back into the café now, and you're going to join me.'

'Am I fuck. I'll be there when the session is done,' he replied.

I walked out onto the mats, and Jay followed.

'What the fuck do you think you're doing? Do you have no respect?' John howled, in a tone of voice that made it sound like we were stomping on his kitten on our way to spray-paint swastikas on his daughter.

'Sensei, you're swearing at a police officer in your own dojo, on your own mats,' I hissed, 'Don't talk to me about respect.'

By now, Jay and I were standing about a metre away from John. I couldn't help but be acutely aware of the 15 blue- and brown-belts standing behind their instructor.

'Get off my mats,' he shouted.

'We will, when you come with us.'

'I'm not coming.'

'Yes, you are.'

'You can't make me.'

'Yes, we can.'

'You think?' he laughed, and took a defensive stance, before shouting something in Korean. The troupe of people behind him took up a pose that I assumed was the start of some sort of training exercise.

'Use your brains,' I said. 'Of course you guys can beat us up. There are only two of us. But if you try, we'll be back, thirty of us. Fifty. A hundred. And you will all go to prison for a significant time. All I want to do is talk to you, John, about what happened to Chris.'

'Put one hand on me, and I'll fuck you up,' John replied.

'Are you preventing me from doing my duty as a police officer?' Jay asked, innocently.

'Damn right I am.'

'Fair enough,' Jay said. He took a step back and reached for his radio.

'Mike Delta receiving four-eight-three?' he transmitted.

'Yeah, go ahead, four-eight-three.'

'We're going to need BSU support at our last assigned. We're being threatened by 16 pyjama-clad ninjas.'

'Received, stand by,' the CAD operator said, before firing off some commands over the airwaves, coordinating our backup.

'In about five minutes we will be joined by a minibus full of riot police,' Jay said, turning to the people behind the instructor. 'I strongly recommend that if any of you don't want to get arrested, you get the hell out of here now.'

Despite loyalty-related protests from their instructor, the group began to peel away, until only two people remained standing behind John.

'Four-eight-three for Mike Delta?' Jay transmitted.

'Go ahead, four-eight-three.'

'Just a quick update: we are now only being threatened by three pyjama-clad ninjas. We chased off most of them already.'

'Received,' came the response after a few seconds. Even through the bad reception, it was clear that the CAD operator was laughing.

'BSU are still on the way,' they added. 'ETA about four minutes.'

With the room more empty, we decided to try to get some talking done.

'There has been an allegation of assault made against you,' Jay said to John.

'Don't be fucking ridiculous,' John said, and briefly glanced at Chris through the glass. 'Look at where you're standing.'

Jay made a point of looking around the room very, very carefully, scanning the walls, as if he were looking for something in the distance.

'England?' he hesitated, after a long pause. 'This is still England, isn't it?'

'What?'

'That's what I thought: definitely England. Which means English law applies.'

'Don't be daft; this is a dojo. People come here to learn how to fight. Sometimes, you get slapped around a little, that's just how it works. You can't get assaulted in a dojo,' John concluded with a triumphant grin haphazardly splayed across his face.

He had walked straight into Jay's trap. I pride myself in knowing the law, but Jay is a walking legal encyclopaedia – especially any part of the law that is linked to use of force. I guess he would have to be: as a former Trojan response officer, he'd spent a significant proportion of his time in the Met with a Taser and Glock strapped to his leg and a MP5 sub-machine gun over his shoulder.

I was rather looking forward to Jay laying the proverbial smackdown on John's deeply flawed understanding of how the law worked.

'Aaaaaactually . . .' Jay started. This was going to be great, I thought, but Jay's monologue was halted before making it out of the starting blocks.

Six officers, dressed top-to-toe in padding, wearing riot helmets, and holding yard-long wooden truncheons and smaller, round defensive shields, had burst through the door. Shoulder to shoulder, they came to stand behind Jay and myself.

'Nice of you guys to join us,' I said. 'We're just having a nice little chat with John, here.'

'Hey,' Jay said, talking to the two remaining pyjamas behind the instructor. 'If you wanted a good excuse to leave, there are six incredibly compelling reasons standing behind me . . .'

The two students' eyes met. They nodded in perfect unison, before sheepishly walking towards the door of the dojo. The riot-clad borough support-unit cops blocked their way.

'It's okay, Nick,' Jay said to the team sergeant, who stepped aside to let the two students past.

'Right, as we were saying,' I started, but Jay interrupted me. There was no way he was going to let me take the lead on this arrest.

'So, John, I've been trying to talk to you as nicely as I can, but you've just been an insufferable troublemaker. You had your chance to talk, but I'm tired of this, and I'm tired of you. So, I'm done chatting, and I'm going to arrest you under suspicion of assaulting Chris. You can explain yourself on tape back at the station instead. You do not have to say anything—'

'It can't be assault!' John tried to interrupt, but Jay continued to read John his rights without skipping a beat.

'. . . when questioned, if you fail to mention something . . .'

'What the fuck? This is bullshit!'

'. . . may be given in evidence.'

'How the hell can it be assault?' John tried again.

'Remember that you are under caution,' Jay said, fulfilling his obligation as the arresting officer.

'You are referring to consent,' Jay said, finally addressing John's protests. 'That consent extends only to activities within the expectations and rules of the activity in question. There is an allegation that you supposedly attacked one of your students, inflicting injuries that are vastly beyond those normally sustained during practice. In addition, he was your student, and you were in charge of him. On top of that, you're a black belt. The very least your students expect of you is that you can keep your cool if they make a mistake. So yes, I have arrested you for assault.'

'Fuck you,' John spat, still standing in his defensive stance.

'Really? Is that really how you're going to play this?' Jay laughed, and took a couple of additional steps back. I followed his lead.

'Right, mate,' I said. 'You have two choices: either, you lay down on your front with your hands on your back so we can handcuff you . . .'

'Fuck off,' John said, revealing a drearily limited vocabulary.

'. . . or we are going to ask the six fine gentlemen behind us to handcuff you for us, and you can add another assault to your custody sheet,' I completed.

John just stood there.

'Fellas, would you mind?' Jay asked, and stepped aside.

In perfect unison, all six officers placed their left legs ahead of their right, dropped their centre of gravity down by bending their knees, lifted their truncheons and held the shields out in front of them. Left foot first, they took a shuffling step towards John. Then another. Then another. Then another. Each shuffle only covered a few inches of ground, but they came in quick succession, and they were gliding along the mat at quite some speed.

John continued his defensive stance for another fraction of a second, before quickly lying down on his front, with his hands behind his back – he must have decided that no amount of black belt was going to stop him from being arrested by six heavily padded officers with truncheons and shields.

'Spread your legs,' Nick, the BSU skipper, commanded.

John did what he was asked.

'Further!'

It was the best possible outcome, really; a suspect on their stomach, legs apart and arms on his back, is essentially incapacitated. There's no way they can jump up or harm any of us without signalling what they are going to do. Just try it: lie face down on the floor, legs wide apart, hands on your back. It's impossible to get up without moving your hands or legs quite a lot – which would give us plenty of time to jump away from you and get our batons ready.

It was certainly a preferable situation than the alternative, which would have been an all-out brawl between six riot police and a load of pyjama-clad martial artists.

Once John was handcuffed, the BSU guys wrapped up his legs with Velcro-and-elastic leg restraints as well. I'm not completely sure that was necessary, but given John's attitude it seemed like a prudent idea.

It was also entirely worth it – just to see the faces of the people in his class, when four of our padded officers carried the instructor out of the dojo, into the waiting caged van.

You don't know what you've got till it's gone

'Patricia Smith? What's her date of birth?' the triage nurse at the other end of the phone line asked.

I answered.

'Nope, sorry, nobody by that name here,' she said, before hanging up.

I sighed, and placed another cross on my sheet of paper. That was the fifth hospital I had called and there was still no trace of Patricia. Or Pat. Or Patty. I had another three hospitals on my list, but I knew I would get the same response.

Patricia is 13 years old. Her mother, Samantha, has three other kids, but for some reason it's always Patricia that ends up in my notebook. This occurrence, I was told by Merlin – a police database that stores information on children who have become known to us for any reason – was the twelfth time Patricia had been reported missing in the past two months.

After rattling through the last three A&E departments without success, I sighed again, got up from my computer and went to my car.

Today, I was operating Mike Delta 79, also known as the 'Misper' car. That's the unimaginatively named 'missing persons' designation. It is, by far, my least favourite job. Not because I don't think it's important to find missing people, but because nine times out of ten, the people who are reported 'missing' aren't, in reality, 'missing' at all. On our borough, more often than not, people have been reported missing almost immediately after they've walked out the front door.

Patricia is a perfect example: she has discovered that her mother gets incredibly embarrassed whenever the police show up at her house. So, she has decided to use us as a tool to 'get back' at Samantha.

I rapped on the window pane next to the door at number 14. Samantha, hearing the sound, came over, but as soon as she spotted the uniform through the frosted glass, I heard her swear. She stumbled around inside for a few moments before she opened the door.

'What is it?' Samantha said. She didn't yet know that Patricia had gone missing. As I opened my mouth to tell her, her mobile phone rang, broadcasting a best-forgotten Lily Allen track into the daylight outside.

'It's the school,' she said, as the penny dropped. She waved me in with her left hand, spun round and flicked the kettle on in one fluid motion. I stepped through the front door into a heavy cloud of marijuana smoke – not the first time at *Casa Smith* – but I was there to find her little daughter, not to arrest her for her smoking habits.

'Aha,' Samantha said into the mobile phone. 'Yeah, I knew you called the police,' she shouted at the person on the other end of the line. 'Do you wanna know how I know? Because they are here already.'

As Samantha rang off, she turned to me.

'So, Patricia walked out of school again,' she said.

The school have a procedure for these things: if a child says they're going to run away, and then vanishes, they call the police first.

I have to admit that I don't really know *for a fact* what they do next, but I suspect they call their own solicitors second, followed by the school's social worker. Then they go and buy some lottery tickets, turn their computers off and on again, contemplate the plot of *Inception* for a while, day-dream about being a rally car driver, think about that fit chick who works in the front office, before they finally get around to calling the parents.

Okay, so I may have made some of that up, but how I managed to receive a call, make eight of my own, pop into a shop to buy a cup of tea, cruise three miles across the borough in lunch-hour traffic and still beat a phone call from the school will have to remain a mystery for another day. When I was young, they at least had the sense to call the parents *first*.

From my Metvest, I dug out an Evidence and Action book and began to take down Patricia's details.

'So, Ms Smith, what was Patricia wearing today?'

I ran through the whole spiel. Did they have any arguments? Did Patricia say she was going anywhere? Did she have her Oyster card with her? How much money did she have on her travel card? Did she have access to any other money? Etc. Etc. Etc.

Missing Persons is an aspect of policing that can be fantastically rewarding – when you are searching for somebody that actually needs finding. The ecstasy on a parent's face when they are reunited with their three-year-old after a few days is absolutely and incomparably priceless. Sadly, most of the time, Missing Persons is absolute, soul-destroying, pointless busywork. Schools and parents seem to think that dialling 101 (or 999 for the particularly clueless) is the first port of call when a kid goes 'missing'. Whatever you do, don't call their friends or their friends' parents. Don't call the school. Don't do a quick stroll down to the local shop to see if they popped out to buy an ice-cream cone. For heaven's sake, don't try calling or texting your kid on their mobile; that would simply make too much sense. Just call the police right away.

Of course – and perhaps this is worst of all, from my (admittedly selfish) standpoint – the catch-22 of my hatred of running the Misper car is that I cannot do a half-arsed job of it. I know some of my colleagues do, but I can't. The thing is, I have terrible luck. The very worst. The day that I decide not to give a Misper investigation my full attention will be the day a five-year-old shows up in hospital, or a three-year-old is kidnapped, or a 13-year-old turns up dead in a skip somewhere. I can't bear the thought. It doesn't remove the fact that we have a Misper car on our borough every day of the week. Whoever is doing the job is always busy for the whole shift. And as you can probably imagine, it's only a worthwhile job once a month, at most.

I left Samantha's and made my way to Patricia's school to take a statement from the teacher who saw her last, but as I pulled out on to the road my radio beeped into action.

'We've just had a report of an incident involving a child. The phone call originated from a phone box outside 12 Lower Street. The woman keeps hanging up and re-dialling 999, sobbing uncontrollably. Can someone please make their way there. Graded I, India.'

I was just around the corner from Lower Street.

'Show Seventy-nine,' I said, and turned my Astra down Lower Street. I didn't even bother with the blues and twos: I know exactly where that phone box is.

But as I pulled up, I saw that there was nobody there.

'Show TOA Seventy-nine,' I barked into my radio. 'No trace, no trace. What's the call, please?'

The operator went quiet for a moment.

'I'll send the CAD to your MDT,' she said.

'CAD UPDATE RECEIVED,' the morose voice from the in-car computer moaned at me. I scanned the CAD, but there was nothing indicating what might have been going on.

'We had reports of a woman's six-year-old daughter being life-less and bleeding profusely. The mother is extremely upset,' the CAD operator said.

'Are there any skippers on their way?' I asked, but it was a silly question really. A potential sudden death involving a child? Every available sergeant would have run to the nearest Panda.

'We've just had another phone call from the same location,' said the CAD operator.

'What?' I mumbled to myself, as I turned around and looked at the phone booth. It was empty. Very, very empty. I stepped out the car and started walking towards the phone booth to make sure, but the absurdity of the situation was daunting; I had a clear view of the thing, and it was definitely, disgustingly and completely empty.

'Mike Delta receiving five-nine-two'.

'Five-nine-two, go ahead'.

'I'm currently looking at the phone box in question; there's nobody there. Nobody in the phone box, nobody near the phone box . . . Nothing. No trace.'

It appeared the 999 computer system was on the fritz, that British Telecom had changed the numbers to the phone booth, or that something Truly Mysterious was going on.

'Stand by, five-nine-two,' the operator shut me up. 'The woman says her daughter is dead.'

A chill ran down my spine.

I can't think of anything worse to hear over the radio.

'We have a partial address,' the operator added. 'She says she is on Jameson Street.'

I swore (lightly, and only under my breath, mind. I am a

professional, after all) and ran back to my car. Blues on. Pedal down. I headed down the road to Jameson Street.

'The house number is given as a hundred and fifteen – one-one-five,' the operator clarified.

I looked out of my window, looking for house numbers. 119. 121. 123. 125.

Bollocks.

I hit the brakes, and brought the car to an abrupt stop. Into reverse. 121. 119. 117. 115. There it was.

'Show TOA Seventy-nine,' I said again, as I leapt out of my car, and propelled myself up the three concrete steps to 115. I knocked on the door.

Nothing.

I knocked harder, and rang all the door bells. There were three of them. Three flats.

'POLICE, OPEN UP,' I said. I had taken my baton out of its holster, and was using the back of it to bang on the heavy wooden door, simultaneously ringing all the doorbells in turn.

An upstairs window opened.

'Can I help you?' The man, in his mid-20s, looked as if he had just woken up.

'Have you heard anything about an acci—' I was cut off by my own radio, clipped to my Metvest and turned to just-a-little-bit-too-loud-for-comfort.

'Cancel, cancel. The address for Jameson Street is a hundred and fifty – one-five-zero. That is, one-five-zero. Not one-one-five.'

Jesus.

'Sorry, sorry, sorry,' I called up to the man. 'Wrong address.'

He shook his head in disbelief and closed the window. I imagine he was probably mumbling 'wanker' at me.

Back to my car.

Car wouldn't start.

Why wasn't it starting?

What the hell?

It finally started. Blues back on. Careening back up the road. I looked to my right. House numbers. House numbers. There. 120. 122. 124. Why was there nobody else here yet? 146. 148. 150. Bingo. I stopped the car in the middle of the road. I left my blues on. Jumped out. Leaned back into the car to press the 'TOA' button on my MDT. I wondered to myself why I just did that. I could have just radioed in my time of arrival. What was wrong with me? I can hear something. Two different types of wailing. A police siren coming closer. A deeply distressed woman moving away from me. Both wailing. I registered that the sound wasn't coming from downstairs and stumbled onto the steps to the ground-floor flat. There was a doorway. A woman. There she was. She was holding a cordless phone in her hands. There wasn't a phone booth in sight.

Whilst I was swearing at a national telephone company in my head, I finally realised that I was stressed. Very stressed. Something about the way this whole job had gone down had really got to me. It happens very rarely, but when it does I'm gripped with a fear of not being in control of myself, as if someone else is remote-controlling me.

There was nothing I wanted more than to get to the woman, and find out what was happening with her child, but I took the time to take a couple of deep breaths. I felt the pulse subside from my ears. That was better. I took another deep breath.

Sometimes, and often for the least predictable reasons, this job really gets to me. I made a mental note to analyse why I felt so helpless. But later. There was no time to dwell.

The woman became a little quieter, and was looking absent-mindedly at the policeman – me – frozen halfway up the concrete steps to her house, who appeared to be doing yoga-style breathing exercises.

'Jesus,' I thought to myself, 'could I look like any more of an idiot if I tried?'

I bounded up the last few steps.

'Miss,' I said.

She turned to me, and I could see her eyes were a mess of tears. Her whole face looked bright red, but despite this, there was something familiar about her.

'Where is your daughter?' I said.

The woman snapped out of her catatonic state and wailed as she stood in the doorway. I wanted to calm her down, but most of all I wanted to find out where her child was. She made a gesture that I took to be a nod, and I walked past her into the house. The whole place was a rancid mess. It suddenly clicked into place: I had been here before, a few years ago. There had been a sudden death here, a drugs overdose, I remembered thinking. I wasn't involved with the case myself; I just dropped off an ICEFLO[36] at the house – but this was definitely the place.

Breaking out of her previous blissfully quiet state of catatonia, the woman threw herself against a wall, squeaking and squealing. I couldn't leave her behind to start looking for the child: she was clearly at risk of causing herself harm.

The phone in her hand was ringing. She picked up.

'I HAVE TO KEEP THE LINE FREE; THEY ARE GOING TO CALL ME BACK,' she shouted into the receiver. It was clearly 999 trying to call her back, but she just rang off immediately.

It seemed that she was so panicked that she was failing to realise

---

[36] Immediate Capture of Evidence for Front Line Officers – or, as most people would call it, a camera. I love that sometimes the acronyms they come up with ('ICEFLO') are the same length as the words they replace ('camera'). Only in the Metropolitan Police . . .

that the people who were calling her were the very people whose call she was waiting for.

Through the doorway I saw a sergeant pull up behind my car and step out along with another of my colleagues.

'What's going on?' the skipper called out, whilst my colleague began the task of calming the woman – who was now on the verge of passing out due to the sheer amount of shouting she was doing.

'I haven't been able to go in yet, skip,' I started. 'I couldn't leave her like this.'

'Go!' he said, turning his attention to the woman, presumably in the hopes of getting some information out of her. I delved further into the house and picked up a groaning sound coming from the far end of the hallway.

In two bounds I made it to where the sound was coming from, and found a young woman lying at the foot of a staircase. She was in her late teens, early twenties. Her arm was quite clearly broken, and she had a slow trickle of blood coming out of her nose.

For a moment, I was dumbfounded by the incredible number of clashing noises all around me. There was a shouting match going on at the top of the stairs. Behind me, through a closed door, a stereo was playing ghastly pop music at full blast. There were sirens outside, and the woman at the front door was still wailing with formidable force.

'And where's this bloody six-year-old?' I muttered to myself.

'Are you okay, miss?' I shouted to the girl at the bottom of the stairs.

She groaned, but didn't seem to be responding to what I was saying. Another police car arrived, and one of my colleagues joined me.

'Call this one in,' I said to him. 'I need to find that kid.'

My colleague was an old sweat[37]. He had been doing this for 20-odd years, and was not one to get flustered about anything except a Liverpool game. He calmly hailed the operator via his PR[38], and started assessing the situation

'. . . I have a female, around twenty years of age, breathing but not responding. It appears she has fallen down a flight of stairs . . .'

At least the woman at the bottom of the stairs was in good hands.

I continued up the stairs, and found at the top six people arguing loudly. There was another woman collapsed on a beanbag chair in what seemed to be a living room.

'Everybody please shut the hell up just for a minute,' I shouted. 'We had a report of an injured child. Where is she?'

I couldn't get through to any of them; in order to make themselves heard over my shouting, they simply increased their own volumes another notch, and the argument continued as before. No one seemed the least bit interested in a uniform showing up, and it struck me that the police might not be an uncommon sight in this house.

I made sure the woman on the beanbag was breathing. There was a small collection of drug-taking paraphernalia on the low table next to the beanbag, and I concluded that she wasn't dead, merely dosed into oblivion. Another colleague joined me upstairs and started calming down the shouting people.

I called in the woman I'd found to Dispatch.

'. . . Female. Mid-thirties. Breathing. Not responding. No visible injuries, but evidence of drug taking. Possible drugs overdose . . .'

I hauled the woman off the beanbag and placed her in the recovery position on the floor.

---

[37] A police officer who's been in the job for a long time; usually a term of endearment.
[38] Personal Radio

'WHERE IS THE GODDAMN CHILD?' I shouted at the arguing group.

The room went quiet, and I realised to my embarrassment that I had let the stress get to me. I hate swearing; there's no excuse for doing so in public, certainly in front of strangers, and especially when I'm in uniform.

'There's no child yet, you fucking spaz,' a girl said, as she patted her belly.

I looked at her. She was heavily pregnant, but sucking on a cigarette nonetheless. I estimated her age to be 17, at the oldest. She blew smoke in my face and her friends took a break in their raging dispute to laugh at her witty riposte. Calling a police officer a spaz: how *droll*.

By now, one of my colleagues had joined me in the living room. He, a little bit calmer than I, saw his chance and seized it: 'We had a phone-call from the lady downstairs, saying her child was dead.'

The room went quiet.

'Yeah, she lost a kid a few years ago,' one of them said. 'Tragic, really.'

'I think she got a little messed up when Cindy fell down the stairs.'

Finally, some information I could use: there was no child and the woman at the bottom of the stairway had a name – Cindy.

'What's Cindy's last name?' I asked.

The mother-to-be (it turned out she had turned 16 not long ago) answered again, and I decided to separate her from the rest of the group to get some more answers.

Who is the woman downstairs? *The pregnant girl's mother.*

Who is woman on the beanbag? *Cindy's sister.*

What had the argument been about? *Whether or not someone had pushed Cindy down the stairs.*

Why hadn't anybody thought to try and help Cindy?

The last question was met with a blank stare, as if she didn't understand it.

The ambulance crews arrived. Cindy was taken to hospital. As was her sister Marsha, the one who was blessed-out on heroin; because we weren't sure whether she had overdosed or not, the paramedics decided to take her into A&E just in case. They asked me to come with them as the continuity officer. I don't think they actually needed me, but I won't pretend I wasn't happy to have an excuse to get out of that house. My adrenaline had been running dangerously high all shift, and a few hours of doing nothing and flirting with nurses at accident and emergency might be just the thing to get my blood pressure back down.

The woman who had made the call about her child was sectioned. It seemed she had been suppressing the death of her daughter for many years. This, combined with sporadic drug misuse, rampant alcoholism, and finding a young, bleeding woman at the bottom of a staircase in the house where her daughter lived, had sent her over the edge.

Cindy escaped with a broken arm, a few fractured ribs and a serious concussion. Her boyfriend was investigated for GBH[39], but CPS[40] resolved that there wasn't enough evidence to charge him with anything. The six different witnesses managed to give eight (!) differing accounts of the events.

Meanwhile, Patricia, the girl I had been searching for at the beginning of my shift, came home of her own accord.

Of course she did. Exactly as she had done the other 20-odd times in the past few months.

---

[39] Technically, an assault where the attacker is intending to cause Grievous Bodily Harm.
[40] Crown Prosecution Service

It turned out that she had just popped to the shop because she was out of cigarettes. She then refused to return to school 'because it is boring'. I later tried to explain to her that she still had to attend, and suggested that she should reconsider her nicotine habit as well, but I got such an incredible bucket-load of attitude in return that I didn't hold very high hopes of this not happening again.

At the end of a day like this, I draw myself a bath, pour myself a pint of Ginger Hare, sit back and wonder what I did to deserve a job like this.

And yet, when I wake up the next day, I'm chomping at the bit to do it all over again.

It occurs to me as I'm writing this that maybe I'm the one who ought to be sectioned . . .

A victim of fraud

'Honey?' my girlfriend called out questioningly, having come home to find my shoes in the hallway. 'Shouldn't you be at work already?'

My eyes, which had been closed in a gentle slumber, were instantly wide open. The title screen of *The Fellowship of the Ring* stared back at me from the television across the room. How long since the film ended? I glanced up at the notoriously inaccurate clock on my wall, before leaping to my feet.

I was still half asleep when I grabbed my jacket and started towards the door.

'I fell asleep on the sofa,' I explained to my girlfriend, and quickly kissed her goodbye.

'There's a parcel for you,' she said, and handed me a large envelope.

'Thanks,' I replied, and was out the door.

As a motorcyclist, I'm normally a huge champion of ATGATT – All The Gear, All The Time – but in this case, there simply wasn't time. I was already half an hour into my shift, and I had a ten-minute ride between me and the police station. My phone rang – before even looking I knew it was the shift sergeant.

I answered.

'Sorry, sarge – I fell asleep – about to jump on the bike – be there in five,' I shouted, stringing my words together unintelligibly, as I violently tried to force my left foot into my right motorbike boot.

'Make it fifteen minutes, Matt, and get here in one piece without a speeding ticket,' the skipper replied, sensibly.

'Yes, yes,' I answered, already slipping into my on-duty radio protocol.

When you are transmitting on the police radios, the first half-second of voice is sometimes cut off, so for short messages you repeat yourself to ensure you're being heard. During a car chase, it's never 'left', always 'left, left'. When you're confirming something, it's either 'affirmative' or 'yes, yes'. I've even heard a motorbike copper transmit 'oh shit, oh shit'.

I made it to work, and discovered that all the cars had gone out already and the front office was staffed, so there wasn't a lot I could do. I decided to stop in on Custody to say hello to the skippers, before wandering down to the writing room to check my email and deal with any outstanding CRIS[41] messages.

As I made it to the writing room, I found myself face-to-face with a couple of the Scene of Crime Officers[42]. I greeted them with a wave, and as I did, discovered I that the envelope from that morning was still tucked in my pocket.

Taking a seat at one of the few spare computers, I opened the envelope. As I peeked inside, I remembered that I had ordered some new equipment: four very fast, very expensive memory cards for my video camera. Excellent; it had taken the best part of a month for them to arrive.

---

[41] Crime Reporting Information System: the computer system where we log all criminal incidences. When you report a crime and you're given a Crime Reference number, it has been issued by our CRIS system.

[42] SOCO. Like CSI, but more British.

'That's some professional kit you've got there,' one of the Scene of Crime Officers said. I looked up and saw an old friend, Trev.

'Where'd you buy them?' Trev asked.

'EBay – got a great deal.'

'Oh. Better make sure they aren't fakes, then.'

I looked down at the cards and shrugged. They looked genuine enough to me. The blister packs were sealed shut. The pack had metallic printing on it. It all looked above board.

'How can I tell?' I asked, and pulled one of the packs out to take a closer look.

'It's not easy,' Trev said. 'But we come across a load of 'em that are forgeries. They look perfectly above board – some of the fakes even find their way into high-end photography stores.'

'So, er, what's the difference between a forged card and a real one?'

As I looked closer at the envelope, I noticed that the parcel was sent from China. That would explain why it took so long for the cards to arrive, but it seemed unfair: the eBay seller had said he was based in London.

'They're generally less reliable, and a hell of a lot slower. Sometimes frauds take a 1GB card and change the electronics so your camera thinks it's a 16GB card. The first time you try it, it works, but any photos you write to the card after the first 1GB get overwritten. Other times they are sizes of the same capacity, but they won't be as high quality or the speed as they should be. Sometimes, it can be really hard to tell.'

'Can you have a look?' I asked him. Trev shrugged, nodded, and took one of the cards from me. He peeled it out of the blister pack.

'Looks real enough,' he said. 'Can I look at another one?'

I passed him the whole padded envelope of cards, and he took the next one out of the blister pack. He examined them both closely and compared the packaging. After that he held the cards up next to one another. Suddenly, he made the sharp-intake-of-breath-through-the-teeth sound that should be familiar to anyone who has ever taken their car to a repair shop. It's the sound that comes before they tell you that something expensive is broken and needs to be repaired.

'Hmmm?' I said.

'This isn't looking good, mate,' he said, and handed me the two postage-stamp-sized memory chips. 'Take a close look at 'em, and tell me why they might be fakes.'

Trev turned back to his computer, whilst I inspected the cards.

I looked closely at the connectors, the labels, the cards themselves. I flicked the 'lock' switch to locked and unlocked a few times. As far as I could tell, they were completely identical, and they looked every bit as genuine as you'd expect from an authentic product.

'I give up, man,' I said. 'As far as I can tell, these things are legitimate.'

Trevor turned to me from his computer.

'The serial numbers,' he said, prompting me to re-examine the cards again. I felt pretty dumb, as I still couldn't see anything wrong.

'The two cards are identical,' I told him.

'Mate, if there are serial numbers,' he said, 'there's no way they should be the same, should they? That's kind of the point of a serial number, isn't it?'

I took another look. True enough, the two serial numbers were the same. I opened the last two blister packs as well. Another two cards – again, the same serial numbers.

'I'll be damned,' I said. 'If I had only bought a single card, I would've never known.'

'Yup,' Trevor said. 'They're pretty good at forging stuff, aren't they?'

Since there still wasn't anything useful I could do at the police station, I decided to find out more about my products. I telephoned the UK customer support number for SanDisk listed on the back of the blister packs. I half expected not to be connected.

'Hey,' I said, as someone answered the phone, 'is this SanDisk customer support?'

It was.

Some cheeky bastard had made a very high-quality copy of the memory disks I'd wanted – down to the blister pack, foil printing, hologram and even the official SanDisk contact details

I explained my situation to Gary-the-friendly-phone-support-guy, but there wasn't much he could do. He confirmed that the numbers we thought were serial numbers were, indeed, serial numbers. He agreed that there was no way that two – let alone four – cards should have the same digits.

'That *is* a serial number we recognise,' he said, as I read it out to him. 'But it belongs to a high-speed Compact Flash card, not an SD-sized card.'

Conclusion: I had a set of forged cards, SanDisk wanted nothing to do with them, and I had a load of storage media I couldn't trust with my photos or videos.

Over the next few weeks, I spent several hours trying to get to the bottom of things. I decided to lodge a complaint with eBay. The seller refused to take the cards back 'because they had been opened'; eBay refused to give me a refund because 'I had to prove that the cards were forgeries'; and PayPal helpfully concluded that: 'The claim does not fall under PayPal's definition of significantly not-as-described and does not qualify for a refund. Your claim has been closed as you failed to provide PayPal with the requested documentation.'

It turns out that a sworn report from a Metropolitan Police Scene of Crime Officer isn't enough for PayPal: they needed 'a statement from a professional who is an expert in the field'. The common-sense argument that four cards with identical serial numbers – a number not recognised by SanDisk – couldn't possibly be legitimate, fell on deaf ears. SanDisk were very apologetic about the case, but Gary-the-friendly-phone-support-guy informed me that they would not be able to produce a written statement that the cards were forgeries, as they had a policy not to comment on the matter.

I was, for lack of a better term, up Shit Creek with a broken outboard motor, and without the oars that common sense would have dictated I brought with me when making my way up such an unfortunately polluted waterway.

After a wave of inspiration, I picked up the phone to the fraud investigation unit, but they told me that being defrauded of a couple of hundred quid wasn't really their thing. The fraud division wasn't going to get involved unless I'd lost at least £5,000.

Damn.

I briefly considered ordering another 80 cards from eBay so that I would be above the fraud team's limit, but decided that putting myself at risk of losing five grand just so my Metropolitan Police brethren-in-arms would look into the matter would be a little bit on the extreme side, even for me.

In a last spasm of desperation, I tried to file a claim in the small claims court via Money Claim Online. They eventually issued a judgement, but when the bailiff tried to serve the papers, it turned out that the address I had for my dear friend the fraudster was in a student halls. Because the process had taken so long, school was now out for summer and he'd moved away. Predictably, he hadn't left a forwarding address.

I was at a dead end.

I had pretty much given up hope, when a few days later I happened to be in the pub with a friend of mine. This friend works as a 'researcher' – he has fancy business cards and everything. You would never hear him call himself a private detective, but that's essentially what he is, so for the purpose of his anonymity, let's call him Sam Spade.

'I have an idea,' Sam Spade said when I'd explained the situation. 'Can you send me the raw source of all the emails you've had from this guy? I'll see if I can't dig something up on him.'

I did.

A few days later, Sam asked me to meet him again in the same pub.

'I've got his address,' Sam said, tucking into his pint of Stella.

He explained, with not inconsiderable pride, how he had been able to track down my fraud: a really elaborate process, the details of which I have since forgotten. It included a lot of googling of email addresses, digging and posing as other people.

It transpired that my guy had a company set up in his name. According to the UK registrar of companies, his was registered to a post box company. With a bit of sweet-talking, Sam managed to convince the company to hand over the guy's real name and private address.

'None of this information is admissible in court,' Sam said, refusing resolutely to give any details about *how* he had managed to convince the PO Box company to hand over the address of one of their customers.

'I suppose I might as well go have a chat with the guy,' I said.

'He only lives in Essex,' Sam said, happily egging me on. 'Over in Hempstead, just outside Saffron Walden! I'll come with you if you like,' he added, with a glint in his eyes.

Sam is one of my motorcycling buddies. On our days off, we often head out to Essex; the A- and B-roads in the triangle between Epping, Cambridge and Ipswich are fantastic for a summer's-day ride, playing cat-and-mouse with each other. It's one of the glorious things about riding a powerful motorcycle: even within the speed limits, you still get a thrill as you zip past cars with the wind in your . . . er . . . helmet.

We decided to make a day of it the following weekend: a ride-out punctuated by a confrontation with the scoundrel who had defrauded me of the princely sum of two hundred and fifty Great British Pounds.

The weekend couldn't come around soon enough.

'I've brought a video camera,' Sam said, when we pulled up at the address he had unearthed. He pointed to the kit he had mounted on his supercharged, positively obscene, more-horse-power-than-a-two-wheeled-set-of-transportation-should-ever-have Suzuki.

'Aha?' I asked.

'I'll park my bike so the camera covers the front door, and I'll "accidentally" leave the camera rolling. Don't tell him you're a copper; just confront him. You did bring your memory cards, didn't you?' he asked.

I nodded my reply before taking my helmet off. Since we were on a 'spirited' ride, I was definitely fully ATGATT this time: I was wearing my steel-reinforced motorcycle boots and my leather motorcycle suit. Underneath, I had my chest protector and a turtleback back protector as well. Covered from neck to toes in cowhide and Kevlar, I felt even more secure than I would have in my police-issue Metvest.

Confrontation? No problem.

While Sam repositioned his bike, I grabbed the memory cards, their blister packs and the envelope from the tank bag on my motorcycle.

At the door, I pressed the white button on the frame – a little tune could be heard from inside. Someone opened the door. It was a red-headed man. He was young – I guessed about 20 years old.

'Can I help you?' he asked the leather-clad apparition on his doorstep.

'Maybe you can,' I replied.

'Are you Zhipeng?' I asked, though I had already guessed (correctly) that this young man with his thick Birmingham accent probably wasn't.

'Naw,' he laughed. 'Do I look like a Zhipeng? His English name is Chip. I'll get him for you.'

He turned away from the door, but then turned back quickly, having apparently had an idea.

'Who shall I say is calling?' he asked, casually.

My mind raced. If I said *my* name, Chip might recognise it, and would possibly not come to the door . . .

'I'm Sam Spade,' I answered.

'Right-oh,' the man said, and vanished inside, leaving the door open.

Chip came to the door. He was tall, and from his colossal upper arms it was obvious he spent a larger percentage of his time than I in the gym.

'What do you want?' he asked, with only the slightest trace of a foreign accent; he had obviously been in the UK for a long time.

'Hey,' I began. 'You sold me some memory cards on eBay. They are fakes, and I would like my money back, please.'

There was a long silence. He now knew who I was and what I wanted, but I could see he was still trying to figure out how I found him.

'I don't know what you're talking about,' he said before quickly stepping back and starting to close the door. I moved my foot forward, and placed it in the crack before it closed. As soon as I'd done so, I realised that I'd technically committed burglary, but I wasn't going to let him just shut me out without getting some sort of resolution.

'Get the fuck away from me,' he said, and he opened the door again – only by a couple of inches – before slamming the heavy wooden door shut on my foot. If I had been wearing normal boots – or even my police boots – I'd have broken a couple of toes at least. Fortunately, my motorbike boots are built for brutality: they are designed to keep my feet and ankles safe in case I come off the bike in a crash. I barely even felt it.

Chip opened the door again, and surprised me by pushing me backwards with both his hands against my chest.

'You can't prove anything,' he said, before taking yet another step forward and pushing me again. 'Why don't you piss off before I call the police,' he said.

'Actually,' I replied, with as much calmness as I could muster, 'that sounds like a good idea. Then we can explain to them how you defrauded me of two hundred and fifty pounds. Let's see what they say to that.'

Chip didn't take that very graciously at all.

'Fuck you,' he elocuted.

Then it happened: his arm dropped down, and he took a step back. I had no idea what martial art he was trained in, but I've practiced enough martial arts in my time to recognise a fighting stance.

'Calm down, let's talk about this properly. I obviously know who you are, what you've done and where you live, and I'm not going to leave until you refund my money. There's no need for all of this. Well done you for tricking me out of two hundred and fifty quid,' I said, my voice dripping with sarcasm, 'but just give it back, and I'll be out of your hair; I won't contact you again.'

He shifted his position again. His legs were no longer next to each other; one was slightly behind the other. He had dropped his head down slightly and bent his knees as well.

I knew exactly what was going to happen next, and knew I wasn't going to enjoy it in the slightest.

Chip was signalling his punch. Actually, 'signalling' would be giving him too much credit. He might as well have written, 'I am going to punch you' in elaborately lettered calligraphy on a post-card and handed it to me.

Or, to put it simply, it was brutally obvious that my newfound friend was a better fraudster than he was a fighter.

'You're about to make a very stupid mistake, my friend,' I said to him. Meanwhile, adrenaline was being pumped into my blood-stream, causing everything to drop into a bizarrely familiar slow motion.

I knew we had a video camera pointing at us. I knew everything he was doing was being recorded. If we succeeded in getting a recording of Chip punching me, the plan would be to visit the local police station and have him arrested by the local force for assault. We would have the video and Sam's witness statement as proof. Hopefully, in his interview, Chip would 'fess up to his fraud, and I wouldn't have to explain how I found him. All of this was racing through my head, as Chip was moving himself into position for the now-inevitable punch.

I promise: I had fully intended to let him punch me.

Unfortunately, ten years of jiu-jitsu training wasn't going to disappear that easily. I just couldn't let him reduce my face to a bloody mess. Despite my pledge to take the hit, I felt my body disobey my brain.

A subtle feint to the left and a very fast side-step to the right brought me close to Chip, inside the reach of his blow. He punched with full force, but I was no longer there. His fist had flown past the side of my head and grazed my left ear ever so slightly, but by this point I had already planted the palm of my left hand against his nose rather firmly. Next, my left hand slid down the arm he had tried to punch me with – his right. When it reached his wrist, my right hand came up fast, slapping him across the face. The slap is a 'weakener' – a punch not designed to harm or disable but to confuse. The hit worked as intended: I could feel the arm I was holding relax slightly. The hand I had used to slap Chip with continued its motion down to meet its partner so that I was holding his right wrist with both of my hands and my back was now facing him. For my final move, I turned around, taking a large step backwards with my right leg, and twisting his wrist upside down. Yanking his hand, I brought him off balance.

This was elementary, white-belt jiu-jitsu stuff. You do this particular movement in your very first jitsy class, and I have done it so many times I could do it in my sleep.

The next step in this series of events would be to snap-kick my shin into his face, before breaking his wrist with a quick clockwise jerk, and then fracturing his elbow by stomping on it with my left shin. I decided to hold back. Securing an assault conviction wasn't going to be easy if he hadn't connected a single punch but came away from the altercation with a broken nose, wrist and elbow.

Instead of causing any real damage, I gave his arm a quick yank, and he was flat on his face. I still had his wrist, and I applied enough pressure to notify him that I could break it if I chose to.

I looked up to find Sam standing next to me, pretending to look a little bored. He bowed down and spoke into Chip's ear.

'Hey, asshole. I filmed all of that. We have it on tape that you tried to punch him in the face. Also, he's a police officer, did you know that?'

Chip responded with a half-sigh, half-moan.

'So what's it gonna be, Bruce Lee?' Sam asked.

'I'll pay you! I'll pay you!' Chip said.

I let go of his wrist and took a couple of steps back.

'Go on, then,' I said.

Chip vanished inside the house, and came back out a minute later holding a wad of cash. He counted up £250, and added another £20 to the stack. He held them out to me, but Sam snatched the stack and made a big show of checking each bill, muttering things about forgeries. When he finished, he looked at me and shrugged.

'Looks fine to me,' he said, adding with a grin, 'Even the serial numbers are different.'

'Are you really a cop?' Chip asked, as we turned around to head back to our bikes.

I opened my mouth to tell him the truth, but Sam was quicker: 'I guess you'll never know. Get yourself an honest job instead, eh?'

Later that night, after I'd changed out of my leathers and had a shower, I met Sam for a thank-you pint. As we sat down, he slid a DVD across the table.

'It's the tape from this afternoon,' he said. 'I doubt he'll claim he was assaulted, but you never know.'

Later that night as I was drifting off to sleep, I thought about Sam. He enjoys bending the rules a little bit too much to make a good police officer, but if he ever pulled himself together, he'd make a fantastic partner.

A Day in the life of a special constable

Part 1: Babies don't bounce

Special constables are an interesting breed of police officer: they are ultimately unpaid volunteers, but they contribute at least 200 hours of their time to the police force every year. Many actually do even more hours than that; quite a few help out every Friday and Saturday night, which is amazing – there's no way I would give up my weekends without getting paid.

Specials come in all shapes and sizes – I know of a paramedic, a lawyer, a taxi driver, a couple of students, even a few bankers. Each brings something different to the job – granted, some of them are better police officers than others (indeed, some of them verge on utterly useless) but most are incredibly helpful in our day-to-day policing. Special constables have the same powers as 'Regulars' – fully employed police officers – and they carry the same equipment.

Specials are on a probationary period much like regular police constables. Unlike regular probationers, however, specials can't go out without 'supervision' – they are generally paired with either a more experienced special, a special sergeant, or a constable. Personally, I quite like having another pair of hands with me when I'm out and about, and the skippers know that I'm a relatively patient guy, so I'm frequently paired up with specials in various phases of their training.

'Why do I do this again?' I thought to myself.

It was just after dawn on a misty Tuesday morning. Don't get me wrong, I love my job, but the first early start after four days off still gets to me. Every. Single. Time.

The muted half-conversation and the stingless banter around the room indicates that I'm not the only one contemplating a change of career, or a quick nap in the changing rooms before heading out.

'. . . is Mike Delta five-nine-two and Mike Delta five-one-one-two,' I heard, snapping me out of my introspective daydream.

I engaged the one spider-sense you inevitably develop as a police officer: the ability to rewind conversations in your head. It's weird; you react to your shoulder number almost instinctively, and even if you weren't really paying attention, you will somehow be able to recall the whole discussion without even really trying. The beginning of the skipper's statement had been, 'Today, two-six . . .'

Two-six meant posted on a Panda, which slightly annoyed me because I had been driving the area car, which is more exciting, during most of my last set of shifts. Then I got irritated at my own annoyance, because I knew that on any other day, it wouldn't matter to me what my posting was; as an advanced driver, I would do just as many blue-light runs in a Panda as in the area car. The only real difference would be the kind of jobs we'd be assigned to.

I wasn't familiar with the other shoulder number that had been read out by the skipper, but it was a four-digit number starting with a five, so that meant he or she would be a special constable.

I glanced around the room and switched instinctively into radio mode when I spotted an unfamiliar, and not unattractive, face:

IC1 female, about 20 years old, roughly five-foot-three, wearing a white business shirt with a chequered tie, and what appears to be a Metropolitan Police stab vest. She is armed with a stick and is carrying handcuffs. Spray not seen but assumed present. If I have to make a risk assessment of the woman, it would be high; she is carrying an offensive weapon (a gravity friction-lock baton) and a firearm (technically, the CS gas canisters we are issued with are firearms under section 5 of the Firearms Act 1968). She is also wearing a stab-proof and bullet-resistant vest, which indicates that she is prepared for a confrontation.

I spent a few seconds studying her, until the officer sitting next to her leant back a little, and I got sight of her shoulder number. Three digits: not a special. She must have been a newcomer, or on loan from another team, or perhaps she just fancied sitting in on our briefing.

When the skipper had finished, I bolted out of the briefing room to secure my favourite car. We'd recently taken delivery of a couple of Ford Focuses (Focii?) with reasonably beefy turbo-diesel engines; but more importantly, more comfortable seats than are found in the Astras. If I'm going to spend eight hours stuck in a motor, I want to sit in one that at least has some semblance of comfort.

As I was doing the full pre-tour-of-duty inspection check, five-one-one-two came up to me.

'Hi,' a young man said, nervously. 'I think I am with you. Is this car two-six?'

'It is today,' I reply. 'Two-six is a call sign, though you won't find it written on the car. I'm Matt,' I said, sticking out my hand. 'What's your name?'

'Uh – hi, Matt. I'm Sydney, but my friends call me Syd,' he said.

'Well, I'm going to be your friend then,' I replied, 'because, no offence, I ain't calling you Sydney.'

'Yeah, my parents have a funny sense of humour. I guess I was named after the city I was conceived in,' he said. 'I'm just glad they didn't get down to business in Scunthorpe.'

We both laughed. I had only known Syd for a minute, but I felt it was safe to assume that I'd get along this guy just fine.

'Do you want a tip, Syd? Write my shoulder number and our call sign on your hand. If you need to radio in, it'll be the first thing you forget, and you'll feel like a right idiot as you're standing there holding the transmit button. I had to do that for the first year or so in this job, until remembering these things finally became second nature.'

'That's a good idea,' he said, and showed me his right hand. He had already written it down.

'Good stuff. But, you should have written it on your left hand,' I said, and flicked the sirens on and off again. Yup, they were working fine. After the checks had been completed, we got in the car and drove off on patrol.

'So, how long have you been a special?' I asked.

'About six months, but I've been really busy at work, so haven't been able to do many shifts. This is my fifth,' he said.

'Your fifth shift?' I replied, and glanced across at Syd. 'And you get put with me? Oh boy, have they made a mistake.'

He looked back, and I spotted something in his eyes. Nerves.

'I kid, I kid!' I said, patting him on the shoulder.

'So what have you done so far? Any arrests?'

'On the first few shifts I was out with other specials,' he said. 'It was interesting, but to be honest, I didn't really get to do anything because the more experienced officers were quicker out of the van every time. I've done a few stops and searches, I suppose, and a ticket for someone who ran a red light. No arrests yet, though.'

'Well, do you know your caution?'

'Yes!' he said, and started reciting it.

'All right, all right, I believe you. So, if you were to arrest me for spray-painting over there . . .' – I nodded towards a wall that had been graffitied so heavily it was hard to tell what its original colour might have been – 'What would you say and do?'

Syd spent the next few minutes reciting his way through the arrest process, without making too many mistakes. Most importantly, he didn't miss out any of the steps.

'Right-oh,' I said, when he finally fell silent. 'Better practise the caution some more, eh? There was only one thing I would have done differently: make sure you don't give him the chance to turn his spray-can on you – get him up against the wall, and straight into handcuffs. It's not much of a weapon, but it would be extremely unpleasant to get a blast of paint in your eyes, and ordering new uniform items because they're covered in paint would also be a pain in the backside. Anyway, we'll see if we can't find you a body today. Keep an ear on your radio and put us up for any jobs you like the sound of. A shoplifter is a nice easy first arrest, so if that comes up, we'll go and deal with it.'

'Seriously? Thanks, dude,' he said.

'Call me dude again, and you'll be walking for the rest of the shift,' I said sternly.

Syd looked over at me and started on an apology.

'*Dude*, lighten up,' I said, with a grin. 'If you can't take a bit of banter, you're not going to last long in this job.'

Changing the subject, I asked him why he'd become a Special.

'I wanted to become a regular,' he said. 'But when I tried to apply, the recruitment office told me they had a full freeze on all recruitment. They said if I wanted to become an officer, the best thing to do would be to become a PCSO or a special. So here I am . . .'

'Good idea. Being "old bill" doesn't suit everybody. It's good to get a feeling for things, I think.'

'It's a bit cheeky, too, though, huh?' he said.

'How do you mean?'

'Well, being a special is a voluntary thing. We get, like, a tenner per shift towards our food and travel expenses, but that's it. So basically, we're paying for our own training, aren't we?'

I thought about that for a moment.

'I suppose so,' I said, 'although for a lot of other jobs, you do a degree, and you have to pay for that too, don't you?'

'Yeah, but in my day job, I work for a bank. We had three months of training, and there's no way I'd have paid for that.'

'Hmm. Yes, I guess that *is* a little cheeky. I did get paid during my training,' I said, 'but that was in the good old days, before the recession. Everything was better.'

'Hey, did you see that?' Syd said.

'See what?'

'That red Corsa. The passenger was holding a baby in her arms.'

'Shall we pull them over?' I asked.

'Sure.'

'Wanna do the talking?'

'Sure.'

'All right then,' I said, and switched on the car's blues, before doing a three-point turn and pointing the car the right way.

The Corsa was ambling along a thinly trafficked road, and the four cars between us quickly pulled over to let our Panda pass. When there was only one car between us remaining, I turned off the flashing disco lighting on the roof.

'Run them,' I said.

Syd started fiddling with the in-car computer, not really seeming to know what he was doing. We weren't in much of a rush, though, so I decided to leave him to it. Eventually he got to the right page and typed in the number plate.

'I didn't get the last group of letters,' he said, after a few seconds' hesitation.

'Echo Romeo Echo,' I replied.

'Thanks.'

The car came back as being insured to a Mr Paulsen, without any other markers on it: not stolen, not suspicious, not used in crime, etc.

'Check him as well,' I said.

Syd copied the driver's details over to the person-check screen, and ran them through the computer as well.

'There's a match,' he said, and hesitated for a moment, 'but I'm not really sure what all of this means.'

I looked at the screen.

'He has been arrested before, and has a marker on him; he is a known drugs user. However, he is not flashing up violence or weapons, which means he hasn't attacked anyone and is not known for carrying weapons. These are all things you need to take into consideration. If he had flashed firearms, for example, we'd have to call in Trojan assistance to pull the car over.'

Syd nodded.

'So how would you assess the risk on this one?' I asked him.

'Well, his car is insured and has a valid MOT, and his arrest was about seven years ago. I'm guessing he's a low risk,' Syd said.

'A low risk? Are you sure?'

Syd fell quiet, realising that there had to be another correct answer of some sort.

'Ah. No!' he said, remembering his OST[43] training, 'He's an *unknown* risk.'

'That's better. For all we know, he's on drugs, or he hates cops,

---

[43] Officer Safety Training

or he may have kidnapped the woman and child. Remember what you were taught in Officer Safety: people are either a high or an unknown risk.'

'Yeah, I should have remembered that. Sorry.'

'Don't beat yourself up about it, and don't apologise! Right, let's wait for a bus stop, and then try to pull them over, so we have a bit of space to work,' I said.

'What about that petrol station over there?'

'Not a bad shout, but it's actually surprisingly hard to get someone to pull over into a petrol station. When I flick my blues on, people usually think we just want to pass,' I explained.

I spotted a bus stop ahead of us and flicked on my blues. The car in front pulled over to the side nearly immediately, and we zipped past. The Corsa took a couple of seconds to notice us, so I briefly turned the sirens on. When I did, they pulled over to the side, and I followed them across. They came to a complete stop, and the driver bounded out of the car, clearly agitated.

'Why are you always picking on me?' he shouted before we had even fully made it out of the car.

Oh dear. I opened my mouth to try to handle the situation, but Syd jumped in.

'Sir, I'm going to need you to calm down,' Syd said.

'Calm down?' he said, facing Syd. 'What the hell are you talking about? This is the third time I've been pulled over this week.'

'What were you pulled over for the previous times?' Syd asked.

A smart move – the man wouldn't have to answer him, of course, but if it turned out he had been stopped for seatbelt-related offences recently, it would change things slightly, and I would have been less inclined to let him off with a warning.

'Drink-driving,' the man said.

'And were you?' Syd replied.

'Of course not! I'm a recovering fucking alcoholic, aren't I? I don't drink or do . . .' He paused briefly, and it seemed like he changed his mind about the sentence that was about to roll out of his mouth, 'anything else any more!'

'I'm sorry about the misunderstanding in those cases, then, sir,' Syd said. 'My dad was an alcoholic, and it was very hard for all of us. I'm glad you're on the wagon. How long have you been dry?'

Syd's questions took the man completely by surprise, and his transformation was astonishing. He had dropped his arms down alongside his body. He was speaking slower. He wasn't shouting any more, and he no longer looked like he might take a swing at us.

'Er . . . just over a year,' he said, after looking Syd up and down. 'A year and two months, to be precise.'

'That's amazing. Keep it up,' Syd said. 'However, that wasn't why we stopped you.'

'Oh?'

'The lady in your passenger seat . . .'

'My wife,' the man interrupted.

'Your wife. She seems to be holding a baby.'

'Yes . . .?'

'Well, that is incredibly dangerous.'

'What are you talking about? Is this about a car seat? We're just on the way to her parents – we left the car seat there last week and we're going to go pick it up,' he said.

'Where is their house?'

'Only a couple of miles up the road.'

'And where do you live?'

'Over there,' he said, and pointed vaguely.

'How far?'

'About five minutes?'

'Would it be possible to talk to you and your wife at the same time just for a moment?'

'Er . . . okay,' he said, and walked to the car, saying something to the woman in the passenger seat. She came out and joined us on the pavement next to the bus stop.

I leaned back against the police car; he seemed to be doing rather well and I was happy to leave him to it.

'Hi. Sorry to make you get out of the car, but there's something I want to talk to you about,' Syd said.

'And what's that, then?' the driver's wife snapped, her voice oozing disdain.

Syd was about to say something, but the man interrupted.

'There's no need to be harsh – he's all right,' he said. I looked over at Syd who glanced back with an almost imperceptible shrug.

'Well, I noticed that you were wearing a seatbelt, but that your baby wasn't,' Syd explained to the woman.

'I was holding on to him,' she interjected. 'I would never let anything happen to him!'

'I understand that, but please hear me out,' Syd said. 'You guys were driving . . . How fast?'

'Thirty miles per hour exactly, officer,' the man said, with an uncertain grin that showed he was stretching the truth a little.

'Okay, thirty miles per hour. I'm not going to give you a citation for excessive speed,' Syd agreed.

He was using all the clichés slightly annoyed police officers use: 'citation'? 'Excessive speed'? The kid's been watching too many episodes of *The Bill*, I thought to myself.

'Let's say your baby weighs a stone. Is that about right?' Syd asked.

'Yeah, he's about fifteen pounds,' the woman replied.

'Let's call it a stone; it makes the maths easier. The problem we have here is that you guys were driving at,' he said, glancing back and forth between them, before placing a comical amount of emphasis on the next word, '*exactly* thirty miles per hour. The problem is that if you are in a crash, you are going to slow down awfully fast. Say, for the sake of argument that you are extremely unlucky and end up in a head-on collision. When that happens, your car goes from exactly thirty miles per hour to exactly zero miles per hour in a very short space of time. Agreed?'

'Yeah, that's about right,' the man said.

I walked around to the car behind the couple to take a quick glance inside; I didn't have any grounds for a search, really, but if I did spot any drug paraphernalia from outside the car, we could search it. It seemed messy, but nothing was immediately visible.

'But I was holding on to him!' the woman stressed – beginning to lose her cool. 'Nothing bad was going to happen to him!!'

'Right, please hear me out,' Syd said, trying to get them back on track.

'Say that you go from thirty miles per hour to zero in the space of about a foot and a half, right? That is an acceleration of about twenty times the earth's gravity. That means that your one-stone baby would go from one stone of weight in your arms, to twenty stone and moving away from you.'

The woman just stared at Syd, but her eyes showed that she was trying to envision holding on to a 20-stone baby.

'I guess what I am asking is: Would you be able to hold on to a twenty-stone object the size of a large watermelon in your arms in the middle of a car crash?'

'I—' she faltered.

'Be honest,' Syd said. 'No, you wouldn't. You wouldn't have a chance. Which means that if you guys had been in a crash, your baby would have flown straight into the windshield. Unlike you, strapped into your seatbelt, he wouldn't have had the benefit of being slowed down gradually. He would be brought to a stop in an inch or less. Then . . .'

Syd was on a roll, and I could tell that he was about to launch into further explanation. He was so caught up in his own discussion, that he hadn't seen how pale the woman had turned. I caught his eye and shook my head at him.

'Right,' Syd said, changing tack. 'You get the picture. Suffice to say that it's unlikely your baby would survive an impact like that.'

The woman turned paler still, as she hugged her child closely. She looked, for a moment, as if she might keel over, but her husband stepped in to put an arm around her.

'So,' Syd continued. 'I'll give you guys a choice. Either you, ma'am, and the baby go for a nice cup of tea over there in that café whilst your husband goes to fetch the baby seat. Or, I'm going to give you a ticket for sixty pounds and three points on your licence, and I'm *still* not going to let you drive off unless the baby is in a child seat.'

The couple looked at each other. The woman nodded, and he shrugged in reply.

'Do you need money?' the man asked his wife. 'For a cuppa?'

'I've got a tenner,' she said. 'Drive carefully.'

Turning to Syd, she said, 'Thank you for explaining, officer. Why don't they explain it like that when you learn how to drive?'

'They kind of do . . .' Syd said. 'But never mind. Just remember; it's your baby's life at stake. Use your seatbelt for you and a car seat for the little one. He's cute; what his name?'

'Jimmy,' she said.

'Hi, Jimmy,' Syd said to the baby, who was fast asleep in his mother's arms.

As the man drove off and the woman made her way across the road to the café, we got back in our car.

'How did I do?' Syd said.

'That was really impressive,' I said. 'I think you're going to do well in this job. You made one mistake, though . . .'

'Should I have given them a ticket? I'm not sure I have the right form on me,' he said.

'No,' I laughed, 'that's up to you; if you'd wanted to we could have held them here until someone brought us the right ticket. Besides, I always carry some in my bag in the boot of the car. Anyway, I think you showed some good discretion there: I think your little speech is going to be more effective than a ticket for them. How did you know all that stuff?'

'It's basic physics,' he said. 'And my driving teacher explained it all to me exactly like that. It kind of stuck with me, you know. What was my mistake?'

'You threatened to ticket the man and give him points, but a seatbelt offence only carries a sixty-pound fine. No points.'

'Seriously? But you get points for talking on your mobile? I'd have thought it should have been the other way around.'

'Yeah, I agree,' I said. 'The only other thing is – I think you dealt with the situation very well – but you should have checked his details. We checked the car and its insurance status, but we don't even know the name of the guy; it may not have been Mr Paulsen at all, and for all you know, the car may have been stolen.'

'Oh shit, do you think so?' he said. 'Why did you let me let them get away then?'

'When you were talking to them, I radioed in and did another check on him via the support channel. Because he has been arrested, they keep things like distinguishing marks on file about him. Did you see anything that might have qualified?'

'He had an Everton tattoo on his forearm?' Syd asked.

'Well spotted. When I did a name-check on Mr Paulsen, they said he had that tattoo. Also, his age looked like it might be okay, and his vague description of "five minutes that way" is roughly where his car is registered. It's not foolproof, of course, but given the circumstances, I was happy that we had the right person and so I didn't want to knock you off your stride. It's worth keeping in mind, though: never assume anything.'

'Never assume anything,' Syd echoed, and looked out of the window.

A call came in over the radio, and we looked at each other.

'A shoplifter,' I said. 'Let's go get you that first arrest.'

He beamed, and pressed the transmit button on his personal radio.

'Show . . .' A long pause followed. I glanced over at Syd and saw his mind racing. He had forgotten what our call sign was. And, given that he was holding his radio with his right hand, he finally understood my earlier remark that he should have written down our call sign on his other hand. He stopped transmitting, lifted the radio away from his face and flipped it upside down so he could see the back of his right hand. He read our call sign, before returning the radio back to his face, and transmitting again.

'Show two-six,' he said.

As he finished his transmission, he produced a pen, and wrote '2-6' on the back of his left hand.

Part 2: There's a first time for everything

'Never assume anything,' Syd said, echoing my sentiment from seconds before.

Syd was a great example of what I would describe as a 'good special constable'. At the time of this story, he was about my age (so, mid-30s, but obviously not looking a day over 27, and dastardly handsome, if I may say so myself) and stood about six foot above sea level. He didn't seem particularly strong or fast, but he seemed to have a well-developed sense of risk aversion. In my car, I like that in an operator. In spite of the odd story of heroics, I have to admit that I prefer to get home in one piece every day. As a police officer, I spend enough time in A&E as it is – usually with prisoners who claim to suffer from 'chest pain', or who experience weird side effects to the drugs they swallowed so that we wouldn't find them. I make a point of wasting as little of my own time in A&E, no matter how cute the doctor might be.

Syd and I had just finished the successful traffic stop described on the previous pages.

The kid had proved he had brains, and showed potential. The one thing he hadn't done so far as a special constable was to complete an arrest. At the beginning of the shift, I had promised to get him his first one if a suitable call came in. Lo and behold, once we had finished our traffic stop, our radios beeped to life: a shoplifter had been detained by staff at a local supermarket.

'Show two-six,' Syd transmitted. We were on our way to his very first arrest . . .

'Do you remember what you need to do?' I checked.

'I think so,' he said, 'but is there a signal I can send you if there's something I'm unsure about? I could pull my ear or something?'

'That could work, if you want to look beyond ridiculous,' I laughed. 'I don't believe in ambiguity, to be honest. How about you just say, "Hey, Delito, what do I do next?" I find that does the trick very well.'

'Won't that look unprofessional?'

'Who cares? I would say that looking unprofessional is far preferable to getting something wrong, so ask away. If things go pear-shaped, I promise to rescue you. Do you want this arrest, or n—?'

'Yes!' Syd said, before I could complete my sentence.

'Yeah, thought so!' I laughed, encouraged by his enthusiasm. 'That's the spirit.'

We parked up directly outside the supermarket, and I turned the rear strobes on; I was parked on a double yellow line, but I really dislike straying too far away from the car.

'Show two-six on location,' Syd transmitted as we climbed out of the Focus. Walking through the front door we were met by a shop detective.

'Hey,' he said, 'I'm Nick Andersen; I'm shop security. Glad you boys could make it. We've got the guy in the break room. He seemed a bit out of it – not really sure what's going on with him.'

'What did he nick?' Syd asked.

'That's the weird thing; I had him on CCTV, and I thought he was acting weird, so I kept an eye on him. Then, at the end of the shop, he went to the cashiers and tried to pay for the goods in his basket, but his card was declined when he got the PIN wrong several times,' Nick said. 'Then, he started shouting abuse at the check-out girl, and loaded cans of lager into the pockets of his coat before trying to leave the shop.'

'So, he tried to pay for stuff, then his card was declined, and he took – how many cans of beer?'

'Four in his pockets,' Nick said, 'and one in his hand. He was about to open it as he was leaving the shop, but I walked up and challenged him. I thought I only had to talk to him about his abusive behaviour, to be honest, but then I saw the beers.'

'Hmm. What was the value of the goods?' Syd asked.

'I did a receipt for you,' Nick said, and gave Syd the receipt he'd been holding throughout their conversation.

Syd looked down at the receipt. 'So, five pounds eighty for five cans of beer? How does that work? One quid sixteen per can seems like a weird price.'

I looked at Syd, and so did the store security manager.

'Wait . . .' I said. 'Did you just do that in your head?'

'Yeah,' Syd said, looking slightly surprised. 'It's easy – five goes into five once, so that's a pound, and eighty divided by five is . . . sixteen, isn't it?'

It turned out that the cans of lager had been on a 4-for-£4 deal, and that the fifth can had cost £1.80, bringing the total to £5.80. It took us a minute to work out what the till had done, but we got there in the end. I made a mental note to test Syd's maths skills in more depth.

'I guess even shoplifters get special offers,' Syd quipped. 'So . . . if you steal two things, and they are on a two-for-one deal, do you get charged with one theft, or two?'

I was stumped for the second time in as many minutes.

'Mate, it really doesn't matter if you steal for one pound or sixty pounds or six hundred pounds. The law doesn't say that theft is "the dishonest appropriation of property worth over ten pounds". Do you remember what it says?' I asked him, mostly just to change the topic.

'Yeah. It's, er, the dishonest appropriation of property belonging to another, with the intention of permanently depriving the other of it,' he said, and thought for a moment. 'Or something like that.'

'Something very much like that,' I smiled. 'Shouldn't we be doing some actual arresting? Are you stalling?'

Syd laughed, nervously.

'Seriously, mate, don't worry about it,' I said.

'First arrest, huh?' Nick asked.

'Yes,' Syd confessed.

'Good luck, son,' Nick said, and grabbed the door handle to the break room, pushing it open. The door swung open with a creak. Inside we were met by a defiant-looking young man. He was sitting on a chair behind a table, sipping a can of beer.

'What the hell?' Nick exclaimed, looking at one of the other people in the room. 'Why is he drinking that?'

'Well, he said he had stolen it and was about to get arrested for it, so he might as well enjoy it,' the security guard sitting next to the shoplifter explained.

The absurdity of the situation struck me suddenly, and I couldn't help letting out a laugh. To be fair to the shoplifter, there was a certain logic to it.

'Right,' Syd said. 'Put down that beer.'

The man did as he was told. Syd picked up the can, and poured the rest out into the sink in the corner of the room.

'I'm going to need you to listen to what I am asking this man,' Syd said to the shoplifter, pointing at Nick the shop detective. 'What we are saying concerns you.'

Syd repeated his earlier questions to Nick, who replied exactly as he had before, explaining the course of events.

'Did you hear all of that?' Syd asked. The man sitting at the table nodded.

'Good. Based on what I have been told, I am arresting you for shoplifting, and . . . and . . .' Syd looked over at me, panic-stricken. I nodded encouragingly, but he wasn't able to continue. He looked particularly desperate as he was opening and closing his mouth, trying to find the next words to say.

'What's wrong?' I asked.

'Shoplifting is not a crime!' he said.

'What do you mean?' I said.

'Well, it's been nice knowing you guys,' the shoplifter said to the store staff, and began to rise from chair. 'This fine officer here just said that wot I did ain't a crime, so I'll be on my way, then. Thanks for the beer.'

'You're going nowhere,' Syd barked and the man froze. 'Can I arrest him for shoplifting? What's the crime?' he asked me.

Finally I twigged what he was talking about.

'Ah. Yes. Technically, there is no crime *called* shoplifting, but there's nothing wrong with arresting him for that; everybody knows what you mean. Later on, he'll be charged with making off without payment, under . . .' My brain froze. Balls! Although technically I don't really have to, I take great pride in knowing my wordings, sections, acts and years.

'Er . . .' I said, and after a pause that felt like it had lasted several minutes, I suddenly remembered. 'Section three of the Theft Act of nineteen seventy-eight.'

Crikey, that had been lodged deep in some dark recess of what masquerades as my brain. Embarrassing, considering that this is one of the most common crimes we run into.

'Either way, that's irrelevant for now. He's got to be nicked first,' I concluded.

'What the hell is this?' the shoplifter roared. 'Some kind of ridiculous fucking joke? Where are the hidden cameras, you fucking clowns?'

'Shut it and listen to this officer,' I told him. The man glowered, shifting his eyes between Syd and myself a few times.

'Whatevz,' he said, sinking back into his chair.

'So, I'm arresting you for theft. The arrest is necessary to effect a prompt and effective investigation of the matter,' Syd said, ticking the boxes on one of his forms for grounds (the offence of theft) and necessity (prompt and effective investigation) for the arrest.

'You do not have to say anything, but it may harm your defence if, when questioned, you fail to mention something you later rely on in court,' he continued with the caution. 'Do you understand?'

'You can both fuck off,' the shoplifter said.

Syd nodded in great seriousness, and leaned over his pocket book, speaking as he was writing. 'You – can – both – fuck – off.'

Syd looked up at me, and I tapped my wrist. He nodded, and mouthed an inaudible 'thanks' back to me.

'Time of arrest . . .' Syd said, fishing his phone out of his pocket, 'is fourteen thirty-nine.' He scribbled the time down in his pocket book, as well.

'I'm afraid I'm going to have to search you now,' Syd said, as he straightened up, ready for the section 18 search of the shoplifter. 'Stand up and please empty your pockets on to the table.'

I bit my tongue, not sure that that was such a good idea: there was still a table between us and our prisoner, and I didn't really like the idea of what might be in our shoplifter's pockets. In the end, I decided to speak up.

'Actually, don't do that,' I said. 'Come over here, and stand with your arms spread to the sides, please; we'll do a proper search.'

Syd shrugged, and approached the shoplifter.

'Do you have anything on you that you shouldn't have?' he asked.

'Nah.'

'Do you have anything on you that might hurt me or my colleague?'

'Nope.'

Syd produced a pair of gloves, and started searching the man, whilst I kept a close watch on them both. He found a wallet in the man's pocket, and handed it to me. I took a look inside, but there was no ID.

'What's your name, please?' I asked the man.

'Leonardo DiCaprio,' he said.

'Right. I bet you're Jack Nicholson as well, then, are you?' I asked.

'Sure, if that turns you on, darling,' he said, with a broad grin that revealed a couple of missing teeth.

As Syd ran his hand around the man's trouser lining, his fingers grazed something. He grabbed it, and held it up. It was a small flat-head screwdriver.

'What's this?' Syd asked.

'A loaf of bread,' DiCaprio replied.

'Stop being a smart-arse,' Syd snapped. 'What do you use a screwdriver for?'

'Driving screws?' DiCaprio said, lamely.

'Do you usually carry a screwdriver down the back of your trousers, stuck into your underwear?'

'Only when I have loose nuts,' the man said, and laughed at his own hilarity.

'Give it here a sec,' I said. Syd passed the screwdriver over to me, and I took a close look at it.

It was relatively new, with a hard plastic handle. I put the screwdriver down on the table and took a quick step across to the man, grabbing my handcuffs out of their pouch at the same time. I managed to catch him by surprise, and the cuff ratcheted in place on his right wrist before he had time to react. He immediately yanked down hard.

'Grab him!' I shouted at Syd.

Syd leapt forward and caught hold of the man's arm. He attempted to pull it backwards to meet the man's other hand, but our new friend DiCaprio turned out to be deceptively strong. He resisted fiercely, tugging his body this way and that.

'Hey!' I shouted at the man, 'Stop struggling right now or you're going on the floor.'

He screamed several incoherent sentences loudly enough to bring a couple of nearby shop workers to the break room. Syd was having problems holding on to him.

'Stop struggling NOW,' I shouted, but DiCaprio did exactly the opposite. He arched his back, and put all his power into wrestling his arms back from Syd.

I swore, pulled back and jabbed him sharply in the stomach, aiming roughly for his solar plexus. Immediately he doubled forward and crashed to the floor. Once down, Syd was able to wrench the man's arm behind his back, where his left wrist met his right and clicked into the handcuff. Then, together, we pulled DiCaprio back to his feet.

I pushed him up against a wall. He was breathing heavily.

'Two choices, mate: we can put you back onto the ground and get more officers in here or you can calm the hell down, all right?'

DiCaprio relaxed a little – realising he had lost the fight.

'Fuck off,' he said, making one last stab at rebellion.

Syd took up a position behind the man, and grabbed him firmly. I nodded to him and Syd took his handcuff key off the quick-release holder on his duty belt and double-locked the handcuffs so they were on their tightest setting.

'You all right?' I asked Syd. He nodded his reply, and shrugged, as if to ask, 'What happened then?'

'If you take a close look at that screwdriver, you would have noticed that it has been altered.'

I turned to DiCaprio.

'Why are you carrying a screwdriver?' I asked, repeating Syd's question from a few minutes ago. 'No kidding around. Not in the mood.'

'To fix radios.'

'Really? You fix radios?'

'Yeah.'

'When did you last fix a radio?'

'Er . . . Last week?'

'Were you planning on fixing any radios today?'

'Yes?'

'When?'

'Later today?'

'For whom?'

'A friend of mine. His radio broke.'

'What's his name?'

'Er . . .'

'Where does he live?'

'Er . . .'

'Do you always use a sharpened screwdriver to repair radios?'

'. . .'

'That's what I thought. I suggest you were carrying that thing as a weapon, and that you may have used it as such at some point in the past.'

When it comes to weapons in public, they generally fall into three categories. A 'made offensive weapon' is any weapon that is specifically made to cause harm: swords fall under this category, as do things like throwing stars, guns (although guns are obviously covered by other laws as well), knives designed especially for fighting, knuckle-dusters, etc.

The next category is an 'adapted offensive weapon'; this is any item that has been specifically adapted to be used as a weapon. A large nail with cloth wrapped around it becomes a shiv, for example. Fifty-pence coins that have been sharpened so they can be inserted between your knuckles or thrown, or bottles that have been broken to be used as a stabbing weapon also fall into this category.

The final group are 'intended offensive weapons'. These can be absolutely anything, provided that someone intends to use them to harm somebody else. One particularly bizarre example I encountered was a knitting needle that a 70-odd-year-old lady, who was suffering from paranoia, had held up whilst shouting, 'I will stab you in the throat if you come any closer.' With those words, her intention became clear, and the needles were taken from her and entered in evidence as intended weapons. Of course, it's difficult to prove whether somebody who carries a screwdriver or a corkscrew around with them intends to fix radios, open wine bottles or stab somebody in the eye, but if you carry a screwdriver into a crowded nightclub without being dressed as a workman, I'm probably going to assume the worst and nick you for offensive weapons – unless you have a good and reasonable explanation, of course.

'Syd, re-arrest him for the new offence, and throw in an assault charge for that little fight there as well,' I said.

He looked at me, wide-eyed, shaking his head slowly. He'd frozen.

'Right, DiCaprio, or whatever your name is, I further arrest you for assault, and for being in possession of an article intended to cause injury. You are still under caution,' I snapped.

'Have you got him?' I asked Syd. He nodded.

'Technically,' I said, continuing my pre-tangential sentence, 'it's not just an intended offensive weapon. Since it has been sharpened, it's an adapted offensive weapon. Easier to prove, so that's a bonus.'

I flicked my radio to the support channel.

'Mike Delta receiving five-nine-two?'

'Stand by, five-nine-two, you're in the queue,' came the reply, before the CAD operator returned to dealing with dispatching a couple of cars to another incident in progress. When they finally finished, it was my turn.

'Five-nine-two, are you still on this channel?'

'Yeah, receiving.'

'Go ahead.'

'Have we got space for an adult male in custody, please? Shoplifting, assault, and Off/Weap,' I transmitted.

'Let me check, five-nine-two, stand by.'

They returned a few seconds later: 'Five-nine-two receiving?'

'Go ahead.'

'Yeah, we've got a space reserved for your guest. Need a van?'

'Yes please.'

'On the hurry-up?'

'Yeah, that'd be good, we've had a bit of a struggle with him,' I replied.

A flurry of radio traffic followed, while CAD tracked down an available van. Meanwhile we radioed in some more details: no, we didn't need an ambulance. No, nobody was injured. Yes, Mike Delta five-one-one-two was the arresting officer. No, we weren't sure whom we had arrested, as he had refused to give his name.

The van arrived, and we loaded the prisoner into the cage.

'I'll follow behind in the Panda,' I said to Syd. 'See you there. You stay in the van; keep a close eye on him, all right?'

'Sure thing.'

We arrived at the police station to find a queue of people waiting to be booked into custody – two were being processed inside and a third was in the cage outside, so we decided to leave our prisoner in the cage in the back of the van whilst we waited.

'That all happened very fast,' Syd said, after a long pause.

'Yeah, it usually does. It's quite dangerous to ask someone to empty their pockets. Chances of someone having a gun, for example, are quite low, but not impossible. I'd much rather one of *us* found it, than risk inviting a prisoner to take his own gun out of his pocket.'

'Shit, didn't think of that,' Syd replied.

'No harm done. As it turned out, he probably wouldn't have volunteered that screwdriver anyway. But I'm much happier that you found it than letting him stand there with a sharpened piece of steel in his hands, if you know what I mean.'

'Yeah, definitely . . .'

'Do you know what happens next?' I said.

'We book him into custody?'

'Yeah.'

Part 3: Behind bars

I looked over at Syd. He had just completed his very first arrest – a male shoplifter – and we were waiting outside the custody suite.

It was time to introduce Syd the Special Constable to the dark art of presenting a prisoner to a custody sergeant.

'You're going to take the prisoner through to custody, and you'll have to present him to the custody sergeant,' I explained. 'Then, you'll have to give details of what you arrested him for, and the grounds for your arrest, along with answers to a load of other questions. You'll know all the answers, but just take it easy. This custody skipper is a good guy and he'll help you out.'

Syd shot me a quizzical look.

'Some of them can be complete jerks, and try to catch you out,' I said. 'Quite unprofessional, if you ask me, but it's their call, really; they're the kings of the custody suites, and they have to be sure that only people who need to be detained are placed in the cells.'

'All right,' Syd said.

'Fancy a cup of tea?' I asked.

'I could murder one,' he said.

I flashed Syd a huge, mischievous grin, and saw a look of panic cross his face. Despite this being our first shift together, he could recognise my 'I'm up to something' look as well as anyone.

I left for the cafeteria and returned a couple of minutes later with two freshly brewed mugs of tea. He gratefully accepted one, but then, remembering my grin, asked if I wanted to swap cups with him.

'What do you mean?' I said, innocently.

'Well, I know you're up to something . . . and I don't want to drink it if you've put something in my tea,' he replied.

'Hah, paranoid much?' I asked, and handed over my cup of tea instead, watching him take a sip.

'Of course, maybe I thought you'd demand to swap the mugs, and so I put something in my own mug instead,' I said casually.

He looked at me, mouth half open, before staring at his tea.

'I just want some sodding tea,' he said, suddenly looking exhausted. 'Seriously.'

I laughed.

'Mate, don't worry, both cups are exactly the same,' I said. 'Which really means that both are pretty disappointing, given that they came from the mess hall in a police station . . .'

He smiled, and gratefully tucked into his brew.

A good 20 minutes later, we heard a gruff voice from inside the custody suites. 'Next!'

'You're up,' I said to Syd.

He walked over to the caged van, and let DiCaprio out, leading him into the custody suites.

These suites can be pretty imposing places at the best of times. The custody sergeants sit on a small podium behind Plexiglas walls (people have a nasty habit of assaulting the custody skippers), with computers and banks of CCTV monitors that cover every corner of the room. When we walked in, Syd was met by a pretty harrowing sight indeed, and the real punchline to my little prank.

Syd was about to fall victim to one of the oldest traditions we have in the police force. Whenever you bring in your first arrest, every other officer who isn't busy with something else comes to look at you presenting your first prisoner to the custody sergeant. In my day, you'd complete your booking-in procedure and then go on the lash with your colleagues. It is a rite of passage, and hell, since I was there to help Syd with his first body, I wasn't going to let tradition fall by the wayside.

I've got to hand it to Syd. Even when met with a room full of 30-odd officers, he didn't miss a beat.

'Afternoon, sarge,' he said.

'Good afternoon, constable,' the skipper said. 'What have we here?'

'A prisoner, sarge.'

'Reeeeeally?' the skipper said, his voice so laden with sarcasm I swear I could feel irony-juice filling the custody reception.

'Well, you're in the right place then, aren't you?' the skipper added to much laughter. 'Well . . . Go on.'

'At around fourteen-hundred we received a message over our radio that a shoplifter had been detained at the Central Super Market on the high street,' Syd started. 'When we attended, we heard that a shop security officer had seen this gentleman take several cans of beer and attempt to leave without paying. He was stopped, and detained in a break room. We arrived at about fourteen-fifteen. I questioned the man briefly, and arrested him for shopl—'

Syd swallowed, before proceeding: 'I arrested him for theft. Upon searching him, I found a sharpened screwdriver on his person, and he started resisting. When we were able to handcuff him, I further arrested him for assault and Off/Weap.'

'Off – Weap?' the sarge said. 'And what's that, then?'

'Er. Offensive weapons, sir,' Syd stammered. 'He had, I mean, he . . .'

Syd paused briefly to compose himself, and looked over at me. I gave him a double thumbs up just low enough that the custody skipper couldn't see my hands. Syd smiled, before returning to serious mode and responding to the sergeant.

'Possession of an offensive weapon, sarge. Specifically, an article adapted to cause injury.'

'Good,' the sergeant said, leaning forward to take a closer look at the prisoner.

'So,' he said, 'what was the necessity of the arrest?'

'To facilitate a prompt and effective investigation into these allegations,' Syd said without a pause.

'Very well. You look familiar,' the sarge said to the prisoner. 'What is your name?'

The prisoner remained silent.

'What's his name, officer?' he asked.

'Well . . .' Syd said, and fell quiet. I could see he was blushing.

'He claims to be called Leonardo DiCaprio,' Syd finally responded. The other officers in the room replied with laughter. 'But I have my doubts, sarge.'

'Did he have any ID on him?'

'No, sir.'

'Well, we'll get to the bottom of this. Mr DiCaprio, I am authorising your detention so you can be interviewed on tape about this matter. You will also have one more chance to tell me your real name.'

Again, not-DiCaprio remained silent, merely shrugging and fidgeting.

'DiCaprio,' the skipper said, 'have you taken anything? Drugs?'

More fidgeting.

The custody sergeant turned to me.

'I think Mr DiCaprio here might be under the influence of some type of substance, and to ensure we haven't missed any drugs on his person, I authorise a strip-search of the prisoner at this time.' He took a quick glance at the whiteboard behind him. 'Please use cell M-five to do the search'.

As I led DiCaprio towards the cell, the rest of the team came over and started patting Syd on the back; a few clapped their hands quietly, and he got more than one more thumbs up. The sarge had authorised the detention of Syd's first prisoner, meaning he had passed his test. There was still a lot of work to do, though . . .

Starting with the strip-search.

If you're taken into custody, you're going to be subjected to a thorough search to make sure you don't have anything on you that could be used to hurt yourself or others, or any items that could be evidence in a crime you've committed. There are three different levels of search: a regular search involves a more thorough search than we can do on the street; the next level up is a strip-search, which means that we remove one or more items of clothing from the prisoner; and the top level is an 'intimate search', which is every bit as unpleasant as it sounds for everybody concerned. Luckily, you have to do a special course in order to be authorised to do intimate searches, and I've been able to avoid doing that course so far.

'Right, let's get this search out of the way,' I said to Syd.

Syd had assisted on strip-searches before, so I let him take the lead. First he asked our prisoner to take his sweatshirt off; DiCaprio passed the item to me and I went through all the pockets and the lining. We repeated the procedure for the T-shirt. Next, his shoes and socks. Then his jeans; I checked the linings, pockets and stitching in detail. I found a crumpled-up £5 note that Syd had missed in the first search, but other than that we didn't find anything.

DiCaprio was now standing there just in his boxers; Syd asked him to put his T-shirt back on before taking his boxers off. There's no reason to make someone be completely naked for a strip-search: it's not necessary in order to complete the search, and there's no point in demeaning people. Once DiCaprio had taken his boxers off, Syd handed them to me for a closer inspection. It pains me to report that they should probably have been washed a few weeks earlier. I didn't try, but I'm relatively sure that if I'd placed the boxers on the floor they would have kept their shape and stood up by themselves. Most unglamorous.

Once de-boxered, Syd asked DiCaprio to squat down, turn 180 degrees and squat down again. He then asked DiCaprio to hold his testicles out of the way, and do the same again. We took a good look, and concluded that whilst DiCaprio could most definitely do with learning a few lessons about personal hygiene, he certainly wasn't keeping any drugs clenched between his butt-cheeks.

'Here you go,' Syd said, and gave him his clothes back, minus his sweatshirt and shoelaces. 'I'll be keeping these,' he said, 'or I can cut the cord out of your sweatshirt and take it out, if you like, but it's unlikely you'll be able to get the cord back in there if I do.'

DiCaprio muttered something that sounded like an invite for Syd to do something anatomically unlikely, so we figured he didn't want his sweatshirt cord cut into slices. We placed his £5 note and the items we had taken off him into evidence bags.

'He's clean,' Syd said, as we returned to the custody sergeant.

'Well . . .' I said with a smirk. 'I'm not sure about that. But at least we're pretty confident he doesn't have any drugs on him.'

'Right-oh,' said the sergeant. 'Go play with DNA and Livescan, and go get me some beauty shots of him,' he added, before returning to his telephone call. I overheard him saying something about a detective into the receiver.

Syd and I took DiCaprio through to the room that keeps the Livescan machine. It sounds posh, but really it's just a digital fingerprint scanner hooked up to a central database. It's not very hard to use (unless the prisoner doesn't want to be fingerprinted. It's just about possible to fingerprint somebody against their will, but to do so requires half a dozen officers and generally results in a lot of bruises all round). It's one of the better pieces of kit we have available to us. It took the machine all of 20 seconds to spit out our prisoner's real name and some details; it appears he had, in fact, been arrested before. Jackpot.

I did my best not to react when I saw the result, and we continued taking not-DiCaprio's DNA (a quick cheek swab) and mug shots for the police database and arrest records.

Once we had returned to the custody desk, I signalled for the skipper to look at his screen. The results of the Livescan check would be showing up in front of him. He nodded as if he already knew what the result was going to be, and pressed a few buttons on his computer, before taking Syd aside briefly. The custody skipper was careful about not being overheard. I could not tell for certain what they were talking about, but from the look on Syd's face, I could see it was something rather serious. Once they'd finished their discussion, Syd turned and spoke into his radio.

The custody skipper began to make idle conversation with DiCaprio for a few minutes, about toothache-inducing inane things; I had a feeling he was doing that mostly to stop the prisoner from listening in on Syd's conversation.

A few seconds later, three officers from my team casually strolled into the custody suite, taking up positions all around the custody desk.

'Thank you, Syd,' the skipper said, before turning to DiCaprio.

'The machine you just used, Mr Everett, was a fingerprinting machine. We have positively identified you, so I know who you are. I know that your name is Lee Everett, and this officer here,' he said, pointing to Syd with his hand shaped like a gun, 'has something to tell you. Listen to him carefully.'

Sid took a step forward, and all the other officers surrounding the-man-formerly-known-as-Leonardo-DiCaprio-now-known-to-be-Lee-Everett seemed to tense up and lean forward as well.

'Mr Everett,' Syd began, 'I have heard evidence of an incident that happened on Thursday, where your brother was seriously injured during a vicious assault by an unknown assailant. He has not regained consciousness yet, but witnesses state that you and your brother had had a loud argument only hours before the assault. In light of this, I am further arresting you for the attempted murder of Daniel Everett. You do not have to say anything, but . . .'

As Syd completed the caution, I contemplated what had just happened.

I have to say, I was a little bit envious of Syd. I've been a police officer for quite a few years now, but I've never actually done an arrest for anything quite as serious as attempted murder.

I was keeping a close eye on Lee, who was standing in the middle of the custody suite floor. Five police officers, along with the usual collection of Designated Detention Officers and custody sergeants that mill around in custody, were surrounding him. On hearing the word 'murder' the FME[44] popped out of his office as well, to take a look at our suspect.

When Syd completed his caution, the custody area fell into complete silence. Only the hum of the ventilation system and a distant howl from one of the other prisoners (who, come to think of it, had been screaming the whole time we had been there) was audible.

Finally, the custody skipper broke the silence.

'Right. You should know that every inch of the custody suites are covered in CCTV and audio recording. As this officer just reminded you, everything you say may be given in evidence; that includes the CCTV tapes. I have to ask you a few questions before we move you to your cell, so please approach the desk.'

The skipper nodded at the surplus officers and they left.

Lee meanwhile stood limply, like a hot air balloon that was being slowly deflated. He became a lot more cooperative, answering all the standard questions asked by the custody sergeants. Questions about his welfare (whether he had ever tried to self-harm; whether he had suicidal thoughts; whether he used any medication; whether he wanted to talk to a drugs worker) and that of others (whether he had any dependents, such as kids, or whether anybody might suffer from his being detained), and a whole series of other questions as well. Lee answered each of them with a 'yes' or 'no', signed all the things he needed to sign,

[44] Forensic Medical Examiner

and eventually allowed us to move him to cell M5 – the same one where we had strip-searched him about 45 minutes earlier.

'So, how are you feeling?' I asked Syd, once we were sitting in the writing room doing the reams and reams of paperwork involved with preparing the information for the case progression unit.

'Pretty good. How did I do?' he asked

'How do you think you did?'

'I'm not sure. I was piss nervous. I barely remember any of it all, to be honest.'

I laughed.

'Don't worry, you did really well. A couple of little glitches here and there, but bugger me if it didn't turn out that your very first arrest was one for attempted murder! I've never done a murder arrest before in my life!'

'Seriously?!' Syd asked.

'No! Unless you find someone at the scene, it's usually the BSU[45] that gets used for those arrests,' I said. 'Makes sense, I suppose; when someone knows they may go down for murder, they might feel as if they have nothing to lose, which could make them violent.'

'Ha,' Syd said, and suddenly remembered the sharpened screw-driver. 'Holy shit, do you think that screwdriver might have been the murder weapon?'

'Well, I can tell you for sure that it *isn't* a murder weapon, since his brother isn't *dead*. But either way, you know more than me, mate. I only found out he might be an attempted murder suspect when you arrested him for it!'

'The skipper didn't say anything about the specifics of his injuries, so I don't really know,' Syd said. 'Can we look it up on CRIS[46]?'

---

[45] Borough Support Unit
[46] Crime Reporting Information System

He was asking whether we could look at the case notes for investigation of the assault.

'Answer your own question, my friend,' I said. 'Is the CRIS report relevant to the notes we're writing up?'

'Yeah, of course, I arrested the guy for it!'

'Hmm. Not quite. You arrested him based on information given to you by the custody skipper, and that is what needs to go into your notes.'

'And after I've written my notes?'

'Are you involved in the investigation of the assault?'

'No . . .'

'Well, then, no. I don't want to be an arse, but the computer guys are really strict about stuff like this. If you start poking about in databases around cases you aren't actively working on, you could get in trouble. Everything is logged, and you had best have a really good explanation for why you're looking at a particular case.'

'But . . . I'm really curious now!'

I grinned.

'Me too! Tell you what, write down the CRIS reference number from the custody cover sheet, and then, once we've written up our notes, you can ask the team skipper; tell him you want to learn more, and that you've just made an arrest for attempted murder. He'll tell you whether you can take a peek, or perhaps explain to you how you can find out more. Call me paranoid, but I never go deeper than I absolutely have to for investigations I'm working on.'

I helped Syd write up his reports statements. We also had to go back to the supermarket to get a statement from Nick the shop security guy; to my delight, he had one ready filled in when we got there.

'Wow, I guess you get a lot of shoplifters, eh?' Syd said.

'Yeah, a few. One of the Safer Neighbourhood guys came in here one day and gave me a template we could use, to save us some time and to make their life easier, so we always include the right bits and pieces.'

Syd looked at the A4 sheet in his hand, mumbling as he read: 'Observed a male aged approximately . . . Attempted to pay . . . Card declined . . . Placed goods in pockets . . . Attempted to leave . . .'

Syd looked up at Nick. 'This is fab, thank you! If you wouldn't mind just signing it as well, we'll be on our way!'

After that we had to fill out a simple MG11 witness statement explaining the circumstances and events of the attempted murder arrest.

When the printer next to us woke from its slumber to print out the final versions of our statements, Syd sat back and looked at his iPhone. 'Crap, this arrest took nearly five hours! Is that normal?'

'Some things go a little bit faster once you get used to it. If there's no queue at custody, I can do a shoplifting arrest in a couple of hours or so. Yours took longer because you're not used to the forms, and because you still have to think about how to put together your statements. Don't worry – it'll become second nature, and you'll soon be able to do your witness statements as fast as you can type 'em up. Like anything else, it comes with practice,' I concluded.

We walked through to the custody suite to use the ATR[47] to stamp our statements and other paperwork. Once stamped, we took the paperwork to the stuffy office occupied by the Case Progression Unit, where we handed over the cases. And that was that.

---

[47] Automatic Time Recorder: an automatic stamping machine that is calibrated to only ever stamp the exact time it was used, along with a code for the police station that did the stamping.

'So, what's going to happen next?' Syd asked.

'Well, I don't know about you, but my shift finished about an hour ago, so I think I'm going to the pub, and I'm bringing you with me. We've got to celebrate your first arrest!'

Syd laughed. 'Well, I can't say no to that, but I meant with the guy.'

'Oh. Well, the CPU[48] will be taking over from here. They'll interview Lee on tape and prepare a case. They then hand it over to the CPS[49] to see if they want to prosecute the case. I have a funny feeling that Detective Carson is going to get on him first, though; he's the guy investigating the assault of Lee's brother. Lee will be up in magistrate's court soon, and they'll probably bounce him straight on to Crown court, because I imagine he's going to be charged with at least grievous bodily harm, if not attempted murder or – if his brother dies – *actual* murder. Either way, the punishment for any of those crimes is longer than six months' imprisonment, which is the maximum sentence a magistrate can impose, so it'll be a one-way ticket to Crown court for Mr Everett.'

'That makes sense,' Syd said.

We walked out of the changing rooms into the yard behind the police station, and straight into the arms of ten guys from our response team who burst into applause and cheers.

'Welcome to the team,' said the team skipper. 'Obviously, it's your round. Mine's a lager top.'

---

[48] Case Progression Unit: officers who deal with cases currently in process.
[49] Crown Prosecution Service

A long climb

Pete and I were standing outside a block of flats towards the north end of the borough. Our destination was on the eleventh floor, but sod's law had struck, and of course the lifts were out of order. Of *course*. Why wouldn't they be? With a sigh, we began the long climb.

I started whistling a song, but noticed that Pete didn't join in. He's usually one of the merry ones.

'What's wrong, mate? You're awfully quiet today,' I said to him.

'I had a dog of a shift yesterday,' Pete responded.

'That bad, huh?'

'Yeah, I couldn't sleep last night, to be honest. I'm knackered.'

'Bloody hell. That doesn't sound like you, buddy. What happened?'

'Mate, it was grim.'

'Go on . . .'

'Got sent to a call, right, from a nineteen-year-old chick who was worried about her neighbour.'

'Sudden death?'

'Ha,' Pete said, shaking his head slowly. 'Well, yes, it was, but it was the worst one I've ever been to.'

'Seriously? Worse than the one at the tail-end of last year, where you had to shove your face down a toilet every six minutes?' I laughed.

Pete's face broke, slowly, almost into a smile. He didn't offer a reply to my question.

'I'll just take that as a "Yes, it was worse", then.'

'So, the neighbour was a thirty-odd-year-old lady. When we got there, I could smell death right away, but *she* was fine,' Pete said.

Ah, the smell of death. There's something so primally disgusting and piercing about that smell – I could feel it burrowing its way into my nostrils when Pete mentioned it. I'd happily place my hand on a Bible and swear that I could smell it right there on the stairwell.

'She seemed completely lucid, like there was no problem at all,' Pete said.

'But the smell?'

'She was carrying a baby.'

'Ah noooo . . .' I said, sensing where his story was going.

'Yeah, mate. It was grim.'

'Shit. How long?'

'The baby had maggots crawling all over it. It was horrible. The mother seemed completely oblivious to the fact that her kid must have been dead for at least the best part of a week. Coroner wasn't sure how long.'

I stopped on the landing, leaning a shoulder against a wall. We deal with a lot of deaths in this job, and I've lost my lunch more than a few times as a result. This was the first time I'd felt as if I should play a violin solo just from hearing a story.

'What happened?'

'I called for backup. I'm glad I did, mate – as soon as we said we needed to take the kid off her, she went fucking bananas. She refused to let us take the sprog. She ran inside her flat and tried to fight us off. She ended up cleaving Jake in the arm with a knife.'

'What? Jake? Seriously? How is he?' I asked.

Jake is one of the toughest officers we have – he normally works on the robbery squad, and he's usually the first person to dive head-first into a fight. He's good at it and he likes it, which is lucky because on the robbery squad he gets plenty of opportunities for three-dimensional, technicolor adventures in fisticuffs.

'Eh, you know Jake. He's crazy. Proud of every scar. I'm sure he's chatting up some cute nurse right now, the bastard,' Pete said, smiling sadly.

'Jesus,' I said, not knowing what else to add.

'Anyway, so we had to section her, and ship her baby off to the morgue. Turns out it was probably a cot death or something, but she just continued changing the little boy's clothes and diapers and trying to feed him as if nothing had happened. She was just in complete denial about it all.'

'Dude, that's fucking horrible.'

'Yeah, tell me about it. I'm pretty shook up. It just makes you think about stuff, you know. The woman seemed completely fine when I met her, but it turns out she was probably the craziest person I've ever met.'

'I'm so sorry, mate. Have you spoken to anybody?'

'Just you.'

'I'd give the helpline a bell, buddy. The number's on the wall next to the lockers up on the third floor. Blue poster. Sounds like it may be worth getting it all off your chest to someone who knows what to say.'

Pete shrugged non-committally.

'Seriously, mate,' I said. 'Nobody's going to think less of you for talking to someone. I'm feeling sick just hearing about it, and I wasn't even there. I can't imagine how you feel.'

Pete started walking the last few flights of stairs going up to our next call, but turned before he reached the top.

'You know what was really fucked up?' Pete said.

'Go on?'

'She called NHS Direct, apparently.'

'What?'

'Yeah. She told us, once she calmed down a little, finally. She called NHS Direct and said that her baby wasn't eating properly.'

'Jesus.'

'They told her to go to a doctor, but she decided to wait for a few days. I think, deep down, she knew that the little boy was no more, but she just wanted to put off being told.'

Hearing that completely broke my heart. For a moment, I thought I might cry.

'That is the single saddest thing I've ever heard in my life,' I said.

'Yeah, I know, right? I mean . . . How do you deal with something like that?'

'Well, she's been sectioned, so she's being looked after. Your turn,' I said, and looked up the steps at Pete. 'Seriously, promise me you'll talk to the people? I'll come with you if you like?'

'I really appreciate it, mate,' Pete said.

Climbing up to Pete's level, I hugged him. It seemed like the only useful thing I could do.

'Shall we?' he said, after a short pause.

'Let's do this,' I said, and we finished making our way up the last flight of stairs.

When we arrived at the right apartment, we found ourselves about an inch of cheap wood away from a cacophony of noise and chaos.

'Here goes nothing,' Pete sighed, and knocked on the door . . .

Twisted Sister

To say that there was no response when we knocked would suggest we could hear anything over the racket from inside.

Pete took his handcuffs out of the carrying pouch, and used them to bang again on the door. This, it appeared, was more effective. The shouting and squealing stopped. (Though the barking continued.)

'Who is it?' said a none-too-friendly voice from inside.

'Police, open up,' Pete shouted back, and then awkwardly bolted on a 'please' at the end.

I had to smile – Pete had recently been accused of being too gruff. However, nobody had told him that we'd all been taken aside – as part of the SMT[50] plan to make the police force more approachable – and told individually that we're too gruff and grouchy. It might be true for some of us, but Pete's one of the good guys; I felt a little bit bad that he'd taken the management-induced criticism to heart.

A man – aged around 30 or so – opened the door, but only a tiny bit. He took a quick look at us before worming his way through the gap to join us outside.

[50] Senior Management Team

'I'm surprised you came,' he started.

'You are? What's the problem?' Pete replied.

'It's a complicated story.'

'Not to worry . . . What's your name again?'

'Oh, sorry. I'm Roger Samson. Call me Rodge,' the man replied, and held his hand out for us to shake. We did. As Pete shook the man's hand, I saw a look of recognition – maybe warmth, even – on his face.

'Well, Rod—' Pete started, but then halfway through decided that he was not, under any circumstances, going to call this man 'Rodge'.

'Well, Roger . . .' Pete finished. 'Start at the beginning, and I'm sure we'll get there.'

'Oh. Sure. Well, the problem is that this is my mother's. The woman you can hear shouting inside is my sister. Our mum recently had a stroke and can't really communicate. I don't know how much she understands of what's going on. My sister decided to move into my mother's flat, and she has turned it into a place completely unbecoming of an old lady.'

'How do you mean?'

'She brings men home all the time,' he hesitated. 'I guess I may as well tell you the whole story. My sister has a long history of drug abuse, and she's a working girl.'

He looked from me to Pete and back.

'A prostitute,' he clarified, as if the term 'working girl' was alien to us.

'Okay, well, that's not good,' Pete said. 'How long has your sister been living here?'

'About a year, I think,' Roger replied. 'But I couldn't say for sure.'

'A year, huh? And how long has this been going on?'

'I'm . . . not sure. I just came out of prison, to be honest. Few weeks ago. It's a long story, but I ended up doing some things I regret, and that's over with now. I want to turn over a new leaf; I have a job and everything these days.'

'I'm glad to hear that, Roger,' I said. 'What are you doing?'

'I work at the DIY store down the road. Give people advice about paints and emulsions, all that. It's not very exciting, but it pays the bills. It feels good to finally be doing the right thing, you know?'

'Good on ya,' Pete said genuinely.

Despite the fact that we deal with shady characters every day of every week, it is relatively rare for us to run into people who seem to have genuinely pulled themselves up by their bootstraps and followed the poorly-signposted path down the straight and narrow. I realised then that Pete must have dealt with the 'old' Roger before. In these instances, my reaction is always the same as Pete's – whenever I come across 'regular customers' who I haven't seen in a while, I'll have a quick chat with them to find out how they are getting on. There's one guy in particular, who managed to tear himself loose from a gang following a long stint in prison for an armed robbery that went all shades of wrong. You get to know the regulars quite well after a while. I wouldn't consider them friends by a long stretch, but you do eventually develop a sort of rapport with some of them – almost a fraternal thing, I think. It's sad when we have to arrest them, and it's great when they are doing well.

'Well, when I got out, I went to visit my mum; my sister had been there for a while already. My sister hadn't even realised our mother had had a stroke. I took her to the hospital right away, but the staff said the stroke had happened some time ago.' He shook his head slowly. 'It really hurts me, my mother's face looks as if it's made out of heavy jelly, and the hospital says that most of the effects would have been avoidable if she'd been taken to see a doctor sooner.'

'I'm really sorry to hear that, Roger,' Pete said. 'How did she not know your mum had had a stroke? Isn't that usually pretty obvious?'

'Drugs,' Roger shrugged. 'A lot of drugs. She just doesn't care about much else. It's a shame, she used to be great, but now she's just a wreck. I barely recognise her these days. Haven't seen her smile since I came out of prison.'

'So, what is all the shouting about now?' I asked.

'Well, I . . . I guess, I flushed her stash of heroin down the toilet.'

'Ah. And she was angry about that?' I asked, feeling a little silly about asking such a blatantly obvious question.

'Yes, of course. More importantly, my mother wants my sister out of the house, but she refuses to leave.'

'And you say this is your mother's flat?'

'That's right.'

'Does she own it?'

'No, she rents.'

'But it is her name on the lease?'

'Yeah.'

'And you're completely sure about that?'

'Yeah, I moved her in myself, when my dad died seven years ago.'

'Right. And your mother told your sister that she wants her to leave?'

'Not as such. She can't really speak anymore, so I asked her if she wanted my sister to leave and she nodded,' he said. 'I think she's tried to tell my sister before, as well, but I'm not sure.'

'Right,' I said. 'I'm going to have to talk to your mother, I think.'

'Hang on,' Pete said. 'Can you make sure that dog is locked away?'

'Rita?' Roger laughed. 'She's loud, for sure, but she's a pathetic little yappy-type dog. She won't harm you. Couldn't if she tried.'

'I'd still rather you locked the dog away, if you don't mind.'

'Of course, I'll go do that now,' Roger said, and went back into the house.

'Hey, I don't care how small the dog is,' Pete said. 'They all have pointy teeth and an unhealthy dose of unpredictability.'

Roger popped his head back out of the door: 'Come on in,' he said.

As soon as we stepped into the flat, a young woman came careening out from another room and started shouting at Roger.

'Oh, so you're not man enough to deal with your little sister by yourself, are you?' she screamed, before reaching deep for the worst insults she could think of: 'You impotent fucking bastard. You absolute fucking—'

'Okay, that's enough,' Pete interrupted, stepping forward into the eyeline of the two siblings. 'We don't need that kind of language.'

'Gentlemen, this is Sarah,' Roger said drily.

'Nice to meet you, Sarah,' Pete said.

'Fuck off,' she replied.

'Very nice,' Pete said.

'We need to talk to your mother, if we can,' I said, turning to Roger.

'Well, that will not be possible,' Sarah shouted sarcastically. 'She can't *say* anything!'

'Does she understand stuff?' I asked Roger, ignoring his sister.

'She understands just fine – I think,' Roger replied. 'She nods, shakes her head, communicates with her fingers, writes stuff down. I'm not sure if she really cannot speak, or if she's too shy to because she slurs her words.'

'Fair enough,' Pete said. 'Where is she?'

Roger pointed to a closed door at the end of the narrow, sticky-floored hallway. We walked over, knocked on the door and went inside.

In the room we found a woman, aged around 60. When she spotted our uniforms, she did a little wave with her left hand, before placing it under her cheek. She tried to make it look as if she was just leaning on her hand, but the way she did it made me realise that Roger might have been on to something: she was shy about what the stroke had done to her, and wanted to hide the visual clues from us by covering the affected side of her face.

'Mrs Samson?' I asked.

She nodded.

'Hi. Your son Roger called us. Is it okay if we come in and talk to you for a mom—' The end of my sentence was drowned out by more shouting and screaming from Roger and Sarah.

Pete nudged me forward, and pointed behind him with his thumb. His sign language was clear: I deal with the silent mum; he deals with the shouting offspring.

I took a quick look around. The room was clearly a bedroom. It was simply but tastefully decorated. There was a small green sofa – more like a large chair, really – a coffee table and another chair. On the far wall, there was a small old-fashioned writing desk. Mrs Samson was sitting in front of it, in what looked like a cheap, but rather comfortable, office chair. A single bed was in the corner of the room; there was a curtain drawn around it, perhaps to turn the room into a small sitting room, by hiding the presence of the sleeping furniture. The room was similarly furnished to the rest of the flat but unlike the other areas, it was immaculately clean.

Mrs Samson beckoned and pointed at the sofa-cum-easy-chair. I sat down and faced her. She smiled slightly, and nodded, which I took to be encouragement for me to get comfortable.

She turned to the writing desk. When she turned back, she held up a small piece of paper that read 'Tea?' in neat cursive lettering.

'No, thank you, Mrs Samson, I've just come from my lunch

break,' I lied. I would not at all have minded a cup of tea, but I really didn't fancy putting her in a situation where she had to brave her descendants to brew me a cuppa.

She turned away again and came back with a new message. 'How may I help, Officer?' it read.

'Roger says he is your son – is that right?'

She nodded.

'Great. And Sarah – is she your daughter?'

She nodded again, but with a little less enthusiasm this time.

'Do they both live here?'

Shake.

'Just Sarah?'

Nod.

'Have you asked Sarah to leave?'

Nod.

'How long ago did you ask her to leave, Mrs Samson?'

She held up four fingers.

'Four days?'

Shake.

'Weeks?'

Shake.

'Months?'

Nod.

'So, you asked her to leave here about four months ago. Did you ask her again later?'

Nod.

'How many times?'

She removed her left hand from her face, and wiggled all her fingers at me for a while.

'Many times?'

She nodded again, and nestled the left side of her face back onto her hand.

'More than ten times?'

She nodded with great enthusiasm and made a sound. It sounded like she said 'Many'.

'Many more than ten times?'

Nod.

'Right. And it is correct that it is your name on the lease of this flat?'

Nod.

'How long have you been living here, Mrs Samson?'

She held up three fingers, then four more.

'Thirty-four years?'

Shake.

Not thirty-four years.

I had to think for a few seconds what three fingers, then four fingers might mean. Suddenly, I understood; she didn't want to remove her hand from her face again.

'Seven years?'

Nod.

'And your daughter, how long has she been here?'

Three fingers, then three again.

'Six,' I said. 'Months?'

Nod.

'Okay, so your daughter has been here for six months, but you've been wanting her to move out for about four, is that right?'

Nod.

'Did you invite her to come live here?'

Shake.

'So she just moved in?'

Nod.

'Did you give her a key?'

She turned her head at an angle.

'Did you lend her a key, and she made a copy of it?'

174

Nod.

'Without asking you first?'

Nod-nod.

'Okay. What about your son, does he live here?'

Shake.

'When your daughter moves out, will your son move in?'

Nod.

'Is that okay with you? Do you want your son here?'

She nodded for a long time, before moving away to her writing desk and starting to write something down for me. When she turned back, she showed me another scrap of paper.

She had written: 'He is a good boy. He looks after me. I cannot live like this.'

'I understand, Mrs Samson,' I said.

I felt quite bad; we're often called to situations like this. A mother's love for her children never completely fades away, but eventually even the most patient of parents realises that there are situations that just simply don't go away. It's incredibly painful for everybody concerned, and at much personal sacrifice many parents keep giving their children 'just one more chance'. It seemed as if Mrs Samson had reached her limit, however.

'My colleague and I are going to remove her from the flat for you. If she comes back, and you don't want her here, you have to promise me you'll call 999 immediately. Even if you can't say anything, please call 999. They will send somebody over to come and help you right away, do you understand?'

She nodded.

'Right. Well, thank you very much for talking with me,' I said. My heart went out to her; she was clearly perfectly lucid and truly frustrated by not being able to speak directly.

She reached out one hand to me, palm down. She kept looking at her hand, rather than at me. I wasn't really sure what she wanted, but I leaned forward and took her hand. When I did, she looked up, eyes meeting mine.

'Thank you,' she said. The words were slurred to the point of being unrecognisable, but the message was perfectly clear.

'It's my pleasure, Mrs Samson. Really,' I said, and she let go of my hand.

I got up and walked out of the room, where Pete had the two siblings sitting down at opposite ends of the tiny living room. They had chosen seats as far away from each other as was humanly possible, which, in such a small room, wasn't far, so they were sitting at the far edges of their respective seats in an effort to be even further away from each other.

'Sarah, your mother wants you to leave the house,' I said.

'You can't do that! I live here!' she protested immediately.

'Get out, Sarah,' Roger said.

'Would you mind,' Pete snapped. 'Let my colleague deal with this.'

'Whatever,' Roger said, and with it he got up and left the room. He started rummaging around somewhere else in the flat.

'You've been told to leave many times over the past few months,' I said to Sarah. 'And today, you're going.'

'You can't throw me out of here; my toothbrush is here! I live here!'

Between her flawed logic, her twitching, and the fact that she seemed to have problems focusing on us or really comprehending what was going on in the room, I figured she was on drugs.

'Have you taken something?' I asked her.

'I'm not a thief,' she replied.

'You know what he meant,' Pete said.

'None of your business,' she replied.

'Well, it kind of is my business,' Pete said. 'Either way, you're going to leave this house in the next three minutes. Grab your stuff, let's go.'

'But I'm making a sandwich!' she said, and started chewing on the right side of her lower lip.

'Sarah, you're sitting on a sofa, talking to a police officer,' I interjected. 'You are quite obviously not making a sandwich, and you're not going to either. You're going to get your stuff, and leave.'

Right on cue, Roger re-entered the room with a bin liner.

'Here's your stuff,' he said. 'Get out.'

'Is that all of her stuff?' I asked.

'Yeah, I think so,' Roger replied.

Sarah leapt up.

'Where are you going?' Pete asked.

'Sandwich,' she said by way of reply.

'No sandwich,' Pete said. 'Leaving.'

'Sandwich,' she said again, and started walking out of the living room. Pete stepped out into her path, blocking her.

'Do you have anything that is yours in the kitchen?' he asked.

'Tea bags?' she said.

'Anything else?' Pete asked.

'Yeah. Bread.'

'Anything else?'

'A corkscrew.'

'Your fucking corkscrew is already in the bag here,' Roger said, shaking the bin liner so it made a clunking and rattling sound.

'What else do you have here?' Pete said, drawing her attention from Roger back to himself.

She began clutching at straws, latching on to any excuse she could think of to be able to stay in the house just a little bit longer.

'Clothes,' Sarah said.

'Got them,' Roger replied.

'Hairbrush.'

'Yup,' he said.

'Toothbrush?'

Roger just shook the bag in reply.

'Anything else?' Pete asked.

'My money!' Sarah remembered suddenly.

'There was a twenty and some change on the kitchen counter, and another tenner in your room. It's in your jewellery box, in the bag,' Roger said.

Sarah started crying.

'All I want is a fucking sandwich,' she wailed. 'You're not going to send me away hungry, are you?!'

'Look,' Pete said. 'You've got all your stuff, and we've run out of time. You're going to leave.'

'You said five minutes!' she screamed, suddenly very angry.

'I said *three* minutes,' Pete corrected her. 'Not five. And anyway, we've been here for nearly seven, so your time is up. You're going. Now.'

'What about my—'

'Look, you're just wasting everybody's time now. Either you take your stuff and get the hell out of here, or we're going to remove you.'

'You can't make me!' she shouted before throwing herself back into the seat she had just got up from. With her right hand she grabbed a handful of the throw that was covering the sofa, and with her left she took hold of the armrest on the other side.

'Sarah, have you ever been arrested before?' I asked.

'Yeah, so what?' she snapped in return.

'Well, then you probably know there's an easy way and a hard way of doing this,' I said. 'I don't really care which one we take, but it's going to happen now.'

'MY SANDWICH!' she wailed, sobbing and tightening her grip on the armrest and throw.

'You have some money,' I said. 'You can buy stuff to make a sandwich. But now – leaving. Come on.'

I feared we were going to have to drag her out of there in handcuffs, but suddenly she seemed to deflate right in front of us as she simply gave up.

'Whatever. You're fucking pigs, you know that,' she muttered quietly, and got up, slowly, like a teenager that had been told to go to her room, wanting to drag out the inevitable for as long as she could.

She shuffled over to Roger, and snatched the bin liner, giving him an angry look. She took a step back, before dropping the bag and lunging at her brother.

'You bastaaaaaaard!' she howled. She landed a punch, a slap and a kick before Pete managed to intervene, grabbing her by the back of her jeans and dragging her off her brother.

'Will – you – calm – down!' Pete shouted, but Sarah continued to try to tear herself loose in order to attack her brother again.

'Right, sod this,' I said. 'Sarah, I'm arresting you for assault.'

I fished my handcuffs out of their pouch, but she had completely failed to hear me, and had continued kicking Pete and trying to get at Roger. Roger did the only wise thing, which was to shrink away into the hallway and around the corner. Because she was flailing her hands at her brother, it was easy to get one of them into a handcuff, but that didn't stop her from trying to wrench herself loose.

'Take her down,' Pete said to me, before hooking one of his legs around both of hers. I had a firm grasp of the handcuff on her wrist, so when I made two quick steps into the hallway she stumbled and ended up face down on the ground.

She wailed. Understandable – being pulled around by a handcuff can be rather painful. In OST[51], these manoeuvres are referred to as 'Pain Compliance', and with good reason. We use them sparsely, but they're extremely effective when you need to bring a struggling prisoner under control.

Once Sarah was on the floor, I used the rigid handcuffs to move her hand onto her back. Meanwhile, Pete grabbed her other hand, and soon both were tucked neatly away in stainless steel bracelets behind her back.

I finished my arrest procedure by reading her the police caution, along with the reason, grounds and time of arrest. Pete kept her on the floor by placing a knee on the back of her upper arm; whenever she struggled, he put a little more pressure on her arm and she immediately calmed down again.

'Mike Delta receiving two-six,' I transmitted via my radio, referring to our call sign rather than my shoulder number.

'Two-six, go ahead,' came the reply, immediately.

'Still at our last assigned. We've just had to arrest a female for common assault. Do we have any spaces back at the nick?'

'Stand by.'

I looked up at Roger, who was massaging his face with his right hand.

'You all right?'

'I think I put a tooth through my lip when she punched me,' he said.

I took him aside, out of earshot of Sarah.

'Lemme see,' I said.

He moved his hand and grimaced. There was quite a lot of blood in his mouth, but it didn't look like a particularly bad injury.

[51] Officer Safety Training

'At least it doesn't look like you've broken any teeth,' I said. 'Shall I call you an ambulance?'

'Er . . .' he said.

'You don't have to . . . But we do need to take a statement from you about this assault.'

'Is that really necessary?' he asked. 'Arresting her? It's a bit much, isn't it?'

'To be honest, mate,' I dropped my voice so his sister couldn't overhear me. 'This was probably the best outcome. It think it would have taken us at least another half-hour to get her out of here, and then she'd probably have come back, so you'd just have had to call out the police again later. This way, at least she's at the other side of the borough, so perhaps she'll think twice about coming back.'

'Yeah, that makes sense. Do you think we should change the locks, too?'

'Yeah, definitely change the locks,' I said to him just as my radio sprang back into life.

'Two-six receiving Mike Delta,' it announced.

'Go ahead?' I replied, as I nodded to Roger.

'We have a space reserved for you at the Hyatt,' the CAD operator said, referring to one of the police stations on the borough that is placed right next to a large hotel.

'Great stuff. Can we get a limo as well?' I replied, stretching the metaphor.

'Sure thing. On the hurry-up?'

'Nah, no rush. We're at the eleventh floor though, and there's no elevator, so we're going to need a bit of extra assistance getting her down. Our customer is a little bit lively.'

'No worries, the limo is triple-crewed today. They're not far off, give them ten minutes.'

'That'll be an hour then, including the walk up the stairs,' I joked.

'Very funny, Delito,' the driver of the caged van cut into our conversation, taking my comment as a slur on his slightly chubby physique.

'Hey! Professionalism, gentlemen,' another voice – the shift sergeant – cut through.

'Received. Sorry, sarge,' I replied. His response was fair enough: it wasn't just us and the CAD operators who were listening in; anybody within earshot of a police officer would have heard that exchange.

'Damn right,' he shot back. 'You're buying the doughnuts tomorrow.'

'And a stick of celery for me, please,' the caged van driver added as we ended the transmission.

'Are you going to stay calm now?' I heard Pete asking Sarah, who was still on the floor.

She nodded and mumbled something.

'I'm going to help you up, and you're going to sit back down on the sofa,' he said. 'But I've had it with your fighting, and if you don't keep your cool, you're going back on the floor, okay?'

She nodded again, and Pete helped her up, leading her to the sofa. She was suddenly as good as gold.

It was slightly annoying that we had to wait for the van crew to arrive, but I didn't fancy my chances in bringing Sarah down ten flights of stairs; it doesn't take a strong or heavy person to drag three people down a flight of concrete steps, and as I've already mentioned, I have a strong preference for keeping myself out of A&E as much as possible.

I took the opportunity to take an MG-11[52] from Roger about the assault, and from Mrs Samson about the events leading to the eviction. For Mrs Samson, I simply dictated the bits that are required

---

[52] MG-11 is the name of the Witness Statement form used in the Met.

on the MG-11 form in the EAB[53]. Usually, I'll fill in people's MG-11s for them whilst they dictate, to ensure it's all in unambiguous language, but in Mrs Samson's case, I left her to write down the rest of her statement herself.

After about 20 minutes, the three extra officers arrived and we were able to take Sarah down to the caged van without incident. We spent a painful hour and a half at custody getting all her property booked in properly. It's usually pretty straightforward, but it rapidly turns into a rather long procedure of itemising when your prisoner is carrying a plastic bag containing everything she owns, and insists on itemising each individual item of clothing.

When I put three 'pink tops' on the custody skipper's desk, there were loud protests.

I'll save you the conversation that followed, but let's just say that I, for one, had no idea that there was a difference between a 'coral tank top', a 'rose camisole' and a 'salmon crop top'. Apparently there *is* – and Sarah had all three garments, but exactly zero 'pink tops'. Go figure.

Once Sarah was fully booked in, searched, fingerprinted, and shuffled into a cell at the station, I slumped into a chair in the writing room, next to Pete.

Whilst I had been locked in a battle over the names and precise colours of various items of clothing, Pete had stepped up and finished all the paperwork, like an absolute champion. We were ready to hand Sarah over to the CPU[54], who would be interviewing her on tape, and taking her through the rest of the process.

---

[53] Evidence and Action Book. A handy little 34-page booklet that has loads of aide-memoires in it, so overworked and slightly stressed police officers can do their jobs better.

[54] Case Progression Unit

'I'm knackered,' Pete said, half-sitting, half-lying in a creaky old office chair.

'Me and all,' I said, and closed my eyes for a moment. 'Please tell me the shift is over.'

'Actually,' Pete said, 'we've been relieved. The night shift took over and the skipper has let us off the hook.'

Awesome.

'Do you want some moral assistance and do that phone call we talked about now?' I asked, referring to the call to the counsellor I'd advised him to make after the particularly tragic sudden death case.

'You know, I had completely forgotten about all of that,' Pete said, looking pensive. 'Nothing like evicting a druggie from her own mother's house to get your mind of stuff, I suppose.'

'Well, in that case . . .' I said, giving Pete an easy way to get off the hook, 'Pub?'

'You know,' Pete grinned, 'I think that's the best idea I've heard since the *last* time someone suggested going to the pub.'

We walked over to the alehouse down the road from the police station, and drank all the beer.

An irate customer

I had just attended a stabbing incident that had gone terribly awry. We had been forced to shut down a road and call in the cavalry to help secure evidence. It had been a bloody intensive couple of hours and I was exhausted. The area was crawling with people: a couple of PCSOs[55] were stopping people from crossing the police line on the pavement, a load of SOCOs[56] were doing their thing gathering evidence, the traffic lads were directing traffic, and I was just standing by the side of the road, shattered, not much good to anyone.

I surveyed the scene. A patch of blood on the road. Blue flashing lights everywhere, interspersed with the odd flashbulb going off as the SOCOs took photos.

When somebody has been stabbed, the CPS[57] will usually try to push for an 'attempted murder' conviction. In this case, since the victim was still in intensive care in the hospital, we didn't know whether he was going to make it – if he died, it would be a murder charge (if and when we found whoever did this). Needless

[55] Police Community Support Officers
[56] Scene of Crime Officers
[57] Crown Prosecution Service

to say, if we want to try to make a murder charge stick, we need to make sure that we get every little shred of evidence we can find – every scrap of fabric, everything an assailant may have dropped, and analyse every drop of blood we can find. As such, the SOCOs get the scene to themselves for however long they want, and the road will remain closed for as long as they want.

To a bystander, the scene must have looked like utter chaos, but to me it was different. Indeed, I felt Zen-like: there was nothing I could do at that moment. The victim was no longer considered to be in critical condition. I was about four hours into overtime pay, and everything was 'okay'.

As always, it was just when I thought everything was going so well that it happened: I heard a lot of shouting and the familiar sound of someone trying to calm somebody else down. Since I didn't have anything better to do, I walked over to see what was going on.

A man was standing half out of his car: one foot in the footwell of the vehicle, one on the road. He was leaning over his car door, shouting loudly at a PCSO.

'Fuck you – you don't have any power over me. I'm running late, and I demand to be told what the fuck is going on here?'

'Please calm down, sir, there has been an assault, and we are trying to find out—'

'I don't give a fuck about your fucking assault. There's not even an ambulance here anymore! When are you going to open the fucking road? I'm running late!'

The man spotted me as I was about a car-length away.

'Ah! Finally someone with some fucking authority,' he said, before turning to the PCSO: 'Jog on, douchebag.'

'Mate, what's the problem?' I asked him.

'I'm not your fucking mate,' he said.

Now, I'm not actually a big fan of swearing. There's a time

and a place, and the scene of the stabbing of a teenager is *neither*.

'Hey, pipe down. I'm not swearing at you, there's no reason for you to swear at me,' I said, already tired of the guy.

'That prick,' the man said, nodding at the PCSO, 'is trying to stop me from getting to my dinner reservation. I'm already half an hour late. Can I leave the keys for my car with you? I'll walk to Upper Street and get a cab.'

'Umm, no, you can*not* leave your keys with me, and I really don't appreciate you talking to my colleague like that,' I said to him.

It's no secret that PCSOs and police officers occasionally don't see eye to eye, but I'm generally a big fan of them. This one in particular I knew quite well: he's smart, hard-working, and became a PCSO as a stepping stone to becoming a police officer. He's definitely one of the good guys.

'You have no fucking idea who I am, do you? I know your inspector, you know!'

'I don't really care who you know,' I said. 'We've had a stabbing, and a fifteen-year-old boy might be dying as you stand here insulting me. Show some respect.'

With that, the man stepped fully out of his car. He closed the door and squared up to me.

'What did you say to me?' he said.

'I told you to show some respect. I don't know you, and you don't know me. The only thing I know is that ever since I set eyes on you, you've done nothing but insult my colleague and myself. A kid might be dying, and in order to have a chance of convicting the culprit, we have to do a proper investigation. If that means that we have to keep the road shut for an hour, so be it. In fact, I don't care if we have to keep the road closed for a month; you're not getting through before anyone else. There's an officer over there directing traffic, so you should be through in about twenty minutes at the most.'

'That's unacceptable. I need to get through now. Why don't I just park over there,' he said, and pointed at a bicycle path on the other side of a flower bed.

By now, I was through being patient with him.

'It's a twenty-minute wait. You can wait for twenty minutes. Call the restaurant, explain what happened, I'm sure they will understand. If you drive through that flower bed,' I said, pointing towards the area he indicated he would drive through, 'I'll do you for careless driving and criminal damage.'

I turned around to talk to the PCSO for a second, but the man placed a hand on my shoulder, and turned me around forcibly, so I was facing him again.

'Get. Your. Hands. Off. Me,' I said.

He withdrew quickly, but was still too close for comfort.

'Get in your car, shut up and stop causing a scene.'

'You fucking dickholes are all the same,' he muttered, just loud enough for me and the PCSO to hear.

'Excuse me? What was that? You have exactly three seconds to get your arse back in your car, before I arrest you for a breach of the peace,' I said, and to demonstrate I meant it I took my handcuffs out of their holder.

The cars in front of his started to move. He stared at me for several long seconds; it looked briefly as if he was going to pull back and take a swing at me. Or perhaps I was wishing that he would take a punch at me, because by now I was itching to arrest him.

I leaned forward, my nose nearly touching his.

'Three . . .' I said.

'Two . . .' I made a clicking sound with my handcuffs.

'One . . .'

'Fuck you,' the man finally said, and climbed into his car. As he drove off, he very nearly ran over my foot. The PCSO had run his number plate through CAD[58] and PNC[59], but it had come back clean.

I turned to him: 'You okay?'

He nodded and shrugged.

'What a cock,' he observed.

It was my turn to nod. We walked back to the crime scene together.

---

[58] Computer Aided Dispatch
[59] Police National Computer

Stopping and searching

'We've had a report of a group of six youths fighting with knives in Guy Street Park, descriptions to follow,' the familiar voice of the CAD operator crackled on the radio. He paused to take the details from the 999 call in progress before relaying: 'We have one IC3[60] male, around five foot five, wearing a black hoodie and a red baseball cap. We also have an IC3 male, skinny, around six feet tall, wearing a dark tracksuit with a large Nike logo, and an IC1 male wearing jeans and a red sweater. Several knives have been seen. More descriptions to follow.'

'Show Bravo Alpha one-zero-one,' the skipper transmitted on his radio, signifying that we intended to respond to the call. 'We're a Blunt serial, one plus two plus four.'

In this transmission, the skipper had conveyed to the CAD desk that we were the unit tasked to combat knife crime on the borough at that time, and that there were seven of us: an inspector, two sergeants and four PCs.

'There!' shouted Jim, pointing between two buildings. The driver pulled the carrier to a halt, before throwing it into reverse and backing up so we could take another look. Sure enough,

[60] African / Afro-Caribbean (*see* Identity Codes in the glossary)

someone fitting the description came into view: dark tracksuit, large brand logo, dark skin colour, on a bicycle. He was coming towards us, but when he spotted the huge silver Sprinter van with 'Police' written down the side, he abruptly changed direction.

'Out!' shouted the skipper, and four of us piled through the sliding door at the side of the van. We headed into the council estate, whilst the van left to cut off any escape at the other end of the estate.

As I turned the corner, I was suddenly faced with him. He was talking to someone over a fence. He started when he saw me, but he had stopped his bike with the front wheel sticking through the black metal of the fence and couldn't easily get away. He dismounted the bike and started to walk away from us, quickly, leaving his bike behind.

'Excuse me, mate,' I said after him.

He kept walking.

'You! In the tracksuit! Please stop!' I called.

He pretended not to hear me.

I started running, and my colleagues followed suit. He didn't slow down, but he didn't speed up either, so we easily caught up with him.

'Stand with your arms to your sides,' one of the PCs said, as we surrounded him. 'You are being detained for the purpose of a search; we've had some reports of someone fitting your description—'

He didn't get to finish his well-practised stop-and-search spiel before being interrupted.

'Fits my description? You mean he's black, yeah?' the suspect shot back, and moved one of his arms down from his Jesus-on-the-cross pose.

'Don't move, keep your hands out to your sides,' the PC said, grabbing his arm and moving it so that it pointed straight out to the side again. I then started the search.

'What's your name, mate?' I asked him.

'I ain't your mate, but it's Hakeem,' he replied.

I continued my search.

'Fuck this, man,' Hakeem said suddenly, as if he'd changed his mind about something. I was on his left side, and from the corner of my eye I saw his right arm move towards the pocket of his hoodie.

'DON'T MOVE,' the PC shouted. I used Hakeem's arm – the one I was already holding – to pull him towards me. He was off-balance now, which made it easy for me and the two closest officers to pull him to the ground.

'What is wrong with you?' Hakeem shouted. 'I haven't done nothing!'

He was on the pavement, struggling violently with three police officers on top of him. He barely paused to breathe as he fired off a cavalcade of swearwords that would make a soldier cower in embarrassment. Two of my colleagues were handcuffing him, and I continued the search, while the sergeant stood back to keep an eye on our surroundings and call for additional backup on his radio. This particular council estate was none-too-friendly to police, and he wasn't going to take any risks.

A group of youths, around six or seven strong, came up to us.

'What's this all about? You guys always picking on us, man,' one of the group said.

'Please stay clear,' the sergeant said, but his plea went unheard under the stream of abuse coming from the man we now had in handcuffs, still face down on the pavement. He repeated himself more loudly: 'I said, stay clear.'

'He's clean,' I reported, once I had concluded my search of the man. He only had a wallet on him, no weapons of any kind. I told him to calm down whilst my colleagues helped him to his feet. We decided to leave his handcuffs on until we'd clarified whether he represented a risk or was already wanted by police.

He muttered something about only wanting to give us his ID from his pocket.

The rest of our carrier arrived and the remaining officers joined us. The group that had been gathering was taken aside so we could concentrate on talking to Hakeem.

'Why the hell? There was no need to throw me on the ground like that,' he said, and struggled against his handcuffs.

'Okay, please listen to me,' I said. 'I'll explain everything, but you really do need to listen to me, okay?'

His volley of swearing was ebbing, so I seemed to be getting through to him. Once he'd finally shut his organ for swearword distribution, I continued.

'We had a report of a group of youths fighting with knives, and you fit the description of one of the suspects,' I told him.

'And what was that description? Black man?' Hakeem spat with unveiled contempt.

To be fair, I probably wouldn't have been very happy to be dragged to the ground by police either, so I decided to take the time to explain everything to him: what had just happened and why. 'Well, yes, but also wearing a dark hoodie, like yours.'

'That fits every one of us,' a man from the group, who were now standing a few yards further up the road, shouted. I'd almost forgotten we were performing for an audience. The comment was rewarded with a burst of laughter from his friends. My eyes scanned the group. I recognised a few familiar faces. One of them I believed I had arrested before. A couple I recognised from the gang identification charts on the walls in our briefing room. Others were unfamiliar to me. My attention switched to their clothing; I was unsurprised to find that the man's observation was accurate. Every single one of them was wearing a dark hoodie – some with a logo on the front, some plain.

'The reason we took you to the ground,' I said, turning back to Hakeem, 'is that we had reports of youths fighting with knives. The description we got for one of them was someone of your height and build, and the description of your clothing fit, down to the logo you've got on your hoodie, there.'

Hakeem looked down and shrugged, as I pointed at the logo on this clothing.

'When you went for your pocket,' I continued, 'we couldn't take any chances: we had to assume you were going for your knife, and none of us wanted to get stabbed, so we took you down and put you in handcuffs.'

'It wasn't even me, though,' he fired back. 'This is police brutality, man.'

I sighed, sensing a very, very long night in my immediate future dealing with complaints. I looked at Hakeem. There was something other than hatred shining through his dark eyes, and it inspired me to not give up on him, even though I was aware that he only saw me as 'yet another uniform'. I imagined he was attributing every bad story he had ever heard about a cop to me personally.

'Do you work?' I asked Hakeem.

'What do you mean?' he replied.

'A job. Work. Earning money. Do you work?'

'Yeah, man, I'm an accountant for a commercial laundry firm,' he said, his eyes scanning mine for a reaction.

'Okay – hypothetical scenario. The phone rings at your office. You pick up and an anonymous voice tells you that someone with a black hoodie, a red baseball cap and a knife was just seen entering your building. The next thing you see is that someone with a black hoodie and a red baseball cap enters your office and starts talking aggressively to one of your co-workers?'

'I'd call the police, wouldn't I?'

'I'm glad you said that,' I told Hakeem. 'But what would your assumptions be about this man? Would you be worried if he reached into his pocket?'

'I see what you're doing, blood, but it ain't the same!' he laughed. 'Nobody ever comes into our office with a knife, are you fucking crazy? We're a laundry, chief, use your brains! We ain't got nothin' worth robbing or nothin'!'

'Ah, but you see . . . the streets are *our* office, and that phone call I described to you? That's exactly the phone call we got over our radios. So we're now faced with the situation I told you about: we got a phone call with a description of a person seen half a mile away from here, and when we turn a corner, we find you, and you fit the description.'

'That's bullshit, though; you can't just search me because I fit someone's description – how do you know it's me? I never carry no fucking knife, man . . .'

'I understand that, but see it from our perspective,' I said, as I unlocked the cuffs from behind his back. He moved his hands to the front of his body and started massaging his wrists. 'The only way we have to figure out whether it *was* you is to search you. If you'd had a knife on you, we would have known we could arrest you and figure out whether you were involved with the episode in the park.'

'Yeah, I get you,' he replied. 'Still ain't fair, though. I've been searched like eight times this year, man, it ain't fair.'

'I know what you're saying, but can you imagine why that's happening?'

''Cause I'm black, innit?' he replied.

'I don't think it is because you're black,' I replied. 'Have you noticed much police here on the estate this year?'

'Yeah, of course. You guys are hard to miss, with your flashing lights and all that,' he said nodding to the police van parked not ten feet away. The van's strobes were bathing the estate in an eerie, pale blue glow.

'Do you know why we're here?'

'Yeah, you keep stopping me for no fucking reason, innit?'

'Not you specifically. Do you know why we're stopping anybody at all?'

'Drugs?'

'That's right. This estate is known for the amount of drugs and weapons floating about. Quite a few gangs, too. We want to make this place safe for everybody who lives here, but to do that, we have to deal with the drugs and the gangs.'

'Yeah. My sister was robbed the other day, man, that ain't right.'

'Exactly,' I replied. 'But we can't do anything about that until we do something about the gangs. To do that, we have to try to remove the drugs and weapons from the area. And to do that, we have to search people. We try to search only people we believe to be gang members, but that leaves us with a problem: gang members don't wear a neon saying: "I'm a gang member".'

'I see what you're saying,' Hakeem said.

'What's that?'

'Well, all the gang members are black, innit?' he said, with a lowered voice, keeping his eyes locked on mine, looking for my reaction.

'Well, that's not quite the case – there are quite a few gang members who are white and Asian as well, but yes, many are black'

'And I'm wearing the same clothes as them, so I look dodgy.'

'Hakeem, it's not that you look dodgy, but I think you're thinking in the right direction here. The problem we have is that we can't identify a criminal or a gang member. All we have are statistics, and statistics aren't on your side, in this case. This is an area that has a lot of gang members. Many of them are black, most of them are roughly of your age and wear similar clothes to you.'

'That's fucked up, man,' he concluded.

'You know, you're right. But the thing is, I haven't got a solution for that. I guess one solution would be to leave everybody in this estate alone, but I doubt that would make things any safer for your sister.'

'Man, why don't anybody ever explain all this shit when they search you?' Hakeem asked, with the half-smile of a man who's just solved a puzzle that has been bothering him for a while.

'Y'know, perhaps we should,' I replied.

'So are you saying I should wear a suit?' he asked.

'No, you can wear whatever you want, but unfortunately, given who you are and where you live, you might find yourself targeted more often than others.'

It has been months since this episode happened, but Hakeem's words have been ringing in my ears ever since. He was right, it isn't fair, but I'll be damned if I can think of a way to make it better.

Slowing down for the weekend

We were having one of those freak, unbearably hot summers. The type of summer you desperately long for when the sloppy London winter is doing its damnedest to work its way into your boots, but which, when it happens, you hate just as much as any winter day. To be honest, there aren't many types of weather during which it's nice to be a Metropolitan Police officer – save the odd few days in spring and autumn, perhaps.

Fridays are notorious for all sorts of reasons. Statistically, traffic accidents are more likely to happen on Friday afternoons. Friday evenings following a hot summer day are silly season. People drink way too much, they are dehydrated after a long warm day, and I swear the summer heat brings out the hormones in full force. In my line of work, there's no such thing as a 'slow' Friday, but tonight, all the planets would be in alignment for a perfect storm.

I mention all of this only because it made me happy I was on the early turn, working from 6 a.m. until about 2 p.m. In other words, there was a sliver of a silver lining to sweating like a spoiled kid in a toy store: at least we'd be off duty before it all kicked off later in the evening.

This particular Friday, I was posted with Kim. I've mentioned Kim before, but not stressed yet what a truly formidable woman she is; Kim is my age, but before I'd even finished university she had had two children. There's something profoundly disarming about a 30-odd-year-old rather attractive woman who has perfected the universal 'mum stare'. I saw her use it on a young armed suspect once. The suspect in question was roughly 14 and armed with a knife, but one look from Kim and she put her kitchen knife down, hung her head and apologised, before offering up her arms to be handcuffed – and all of that without saying a single word! She's one of the best police officers I know.

Kim has been married to one of the custody sergeants at our nick for many years. A rocky relationship, I have no doubt, but at the end of the day, there's something deep and genuine between Kim and her husband, Jacob; they seem to have reached a perfect balance of laughing and shouting at each other.

After a particularly spirited fight, Jacob once drunkenly confided to me, 'Kim has this thing she does. She sleeps naked, and when she gets up, she drowsily shakes her hair out of her face, before she grabs her underwear and a pair of jeans. She then forces that amazing arse of hers into a pair of trousers that only just fit. In the process, she jumps up and down and wiggles back and forth. I have to tell you, Matt, the way her breasts move when she does that . . . I could never leave her for that sight alone.'

I've never brought up Jacob's story since, of course, but – curse him – I've never been able to see Kim in quite the same way again. If she were single . . .

Kim and I were doing our usual thing: manning the area car, a lovely BMW 5-Series that is used for general support and fast-response duties. Our end of the borough is a crinkly mess of back roads and one-way systems, so in reality, the Beamer rarely arrives faster than the Astras, but the additional comfort and the feel-good factor of being on the area car makes it a good posting. So far today, we had helped out with a resented stop-and-search that ended up in a couple of arrests for assault on a police officer. We also attended as a second pair of hands on a domestic dispute where two brothers had decided to settle a disagreement with their fists (another pair of assault arrests). Last but not least, we ended up standing around, directing traffic around the site of a particularly nasty traffic accident involving a cyclist and a black cab.

'Two-zero receiving Mike Delta,' my radio murmured.

'Twenty receiving, go ahead,' I replied.

'You're showing green, are you tied up at the moment?' the CAD operator enquired, referring to the fact that our status was set as 'on patrol', which causes our call sign to show up green or 'not deployed' on the CAD software.

'We're just directing traffic around the incident in Chute Street,' I said, as a set of flashing blue lights approached. Reinforcements, in the shape of a traffic patrol car, had just rocked up. I pressed my PTT[61] button again to resume my transmission. 'Looks like traffic just arrived, so I think we can be stood down from this in a couple of minutes. What have you got?'

After we made sure that the traffic guys didn't need us we took off to the next job.

'I'm not really sure what the deal is here,' I said to Kim. 'The operator was saying something about a school, but it's not completely clear what's happening. Can you check the CAD and fill me in?'

Kim looked through the pages that had been sent to our in-car computer and chose bits to read out loud to me.

'I'm not really sure what this is about either, it looks like the 999 operator has been smoking crack rock,' Kim said. 'But I'm pretty sure you were right about the school, although there are three other addresses on this bloody CAD as well. Let's go take a look at the school first.'

---

[61] Push To Talk

When we arrived we were met by one of the teachers who led us to a nurse's office. Inside, a paramedic was finishing up his assessment of a girl from the school.

'You're going to be all right,' the paramedic said to the girl, as we came in, 'but since you've had a knock on the head, we're going to take you to the hospital to make sure. I've got to fill in some paperwork, though, so perhaps you can talk to the officers here first.'

The paramedic looked at me, winked at Kim and went back to his paperwork.

Kim took out her notepad and started questioning the student. It turned out she was 14 years old, her name was Sandra ('my friends call me San. Like Sam, but with an N. There's another Sandra, you see, so people call me San') and she had been in a fight.

'So what happened was that, like, Lateesha was calling me names and I said to stop and then Tiff told her to shut up but Lateesha had already texted Winnie and Sam on her Blackberry, but then Ms King saw her and stopped them from shouting at me but then they sent me a message on Facebook but I didn't get it because I've blocked her and she doesn't know that, but I didn't respond and then she just sent a message to Jim instead and Lateesha really likes Jim but nobody is supposed to know about that and then I said that she really liked Jim and she told me to shut up but then Ms King came back and told me to go to the other end of the schoolyard but she has no right to do that 'cause it's a free country and I refused to go, but then Lateesha went to the loos but I didn't know that was where she was so when I went to the loo they jumped me and I ran out where I bumped into Jim, and Lateesha followed me but Sandra was talking to Jim so—'

It was as if someone had turned on a tap that was spewing an uninterruptable stream of seemingly unconnected words and phrases.

I glanced over at Kim's notebook. She had written 'Sandra McOwen – DOB/06011998', and nothing else. Kim looked up at me, and tried really hard to suppress a smile. She nearly succeeded.

'Hey San, you're going to have to stop there for a moment,' she said. 'You've got to remember that I don't know any of these people; let's start at the beginning, what happened?'

We spent a very long time teasing the full story out of San, and ended up taking a 'good cop, tangent-referee' approach: Kim was the understanding listener, and I had to step in every 24 seconds or so to get San back on topic. We still learnt a lot of 'off-topic' information, such as San's taste in music (she doesn't like dubstep), to her school politics (she was baffled that wearing her necklace wasn't a human right – how dare they take it away from her?), to recent developments in reality TV shows (I would recap, but I fear I'd be showing my age; I had absolutely no idea which shows she was referring to).

The facts, it turned out, could be succinctly summarised as follows: Lateesha is the 18-year-old sister of one of San's classmates. San and Lateesha have an ongoing tiff that flares up at irregular intervals. Today's episode started two days ago, when Lateesha said something about San. San retaliated by *fraping*[62] Lateesha. Lateesha retaliated by gathering her friends in the schoolyard and then beating up San, using her keys and key-rings as a weapon. In the altercation, San was slashed with the keys across her arm and on the face. She then fell to the ground, hitting her head against a bench.

---

[62] Aka Facebook Raping – to change someone else's Facebook status or information without their permission or knowledge. As a general rule, 'fraping' has nothing to do with actual sexual assault. However, because our police crime systems have filters in place, whenever we write 'Facebook rape' in a police report, especially when it refers to victims of crime under the age of 18, it sets off all sorts of extravagant alarm bells over at Scotland Yard. But that, as they say, is a) a story for another day, and b) SEP (Someone Else's Problem).

We had finished taking our statement and were ready to let the paramedic take San to hospital for a more thorough check-up, when San let another morsel of information slip: 'I guess you'll be able to see all about it on YouTube tomorrow anyway.'

'Wait a minute – how would this end up on YouTube?' Kim asked. 'Has that happened before?'

'Yeah, all the time, but then YouTube takes it down again,' San said, her voice betraying more than just a trace of bitterness. 'Not until the whole school has seen it, though.'

'So . . . Someone was filming this?' Kim asked.

San nodded: 'Yeah. Sandra. The other Sandra. She's got a Blackberry and she's always filming shit. She thinks she's Spielberg or summat.'

'Do you know what Sandra's last name is?' Kim asked.

San told her.

'What about her address? Do you know where she lives?'

San did not.

I left the nurse's office and went to find a teacher.

'Hey, we need the address for one of your students,' I said. 'Can you help?'

She referred me to the school office.

'Hey, I'm Matt Delito,' I introduced myself. 'I'm investigating an assault on one of your students, and we urgently need to speak to Sandra Hollywell; could you give me her address?'

'Sorry, we can't give out information about our students,' the lady behind the counter informed me, and nodded firmly. 'Data protection and all that.'

'But . . .' I began to protest, but the lady leant forward, as if anticipating my argument.

'We. Can't. Give. Out. Information. About. Our. Students,' she said, with the tone usually reserved for only the slowest of children.

I went back to the nurse's office where Kim was showing San something on her mobile phone.

'I think we have her address,' Kim said. It turned out the two Sandras were friends on Facebook, and that Sandra Two, the bully, had just checked in at 'home'. Her address had popped up on the map application; that's all we needed.

We left San in the care of the paramedic.

'You know what we're going to have to do, don't you?' Kim said to me, as she shoved her notebook back into her stab vest.

I nodded, curtly. We were going to have to find Sandra and confiscate her mobile phone as evidence; assault is serious business, and the video might be crucial in securing a charge against Lateesha. However, if Sandra somehow realised the importance or severity of the film she had on her phone, she might delete it, which would leave us with nothing.

'Right, you've got the address?' I asked.

Kim nodded.

'Right-oh. Let's go deal with this bully, then,' I said.

As we were leaving the room, I turned quickly to San. 'Please, don't tell any of your classmates that you've spoken to the police yet. We need to find Sandra, and it's best if she doesn't know she's about to get a visit from us.'

San was bouncing up and down in excitement.

'It's just like *CSI!*' she said, with a huge smile on her face.

'Er,' Kim said, looking over at me briefly. 'Yes. *Exactly* like that.'

We climbed back into the BMW, and Kim started typing the address into the car's Mobile Data Terminal.

When we arrived at the estate at which she'd 'checked' herself into, we saw a girl who fit Sandra's description outside.

'Hi there,' Kim said to the girl, who was typing away on a mobile phone.

'Hey,' she said, without even looking up.

Kim stopped right in front of her. When the girl finally registered Kim, and her uniform, she nearly dropped her phone.

'Uh, is anything wrong?' she asked.

'Nothing to worry about,' said Kim. 'I just want to ask you a few questions, is all. Are you Sandra?'

As soon as the name was mentioned, the girl's eyes darted back and forth between me and Kim. She remained silent.

'Are you Sandra?' Kim asked again, positioning herself off to one side. I stood on the other side, just in case she decided to make a run for it.

'Maaaaaaybe,' she said smartly.

In the process, she made our job a lot harder – given that she hadn't committed a crime per se, there wasn't much we could do to make her to talk to us. We wouldn't be able to arrest her, given that we didn't have any grounds or reason for arrest.

'Am I under arrest?' the girl asked.

'No! Not at all!' Kim smiled. 'You have nothing to worry about, but something happened at Sandra's school today, so we need to talk to her.'

'I don't know anything,' the girl said, and started walking towards the gate leaving the estate. I looked over at Kim and she looked back, shrugging.

Another girl came out of a building, and she shouted out to the girl who was about to leave.

'Hey! Where are you going?'

'These cops are here for you,' she shouted back, and kept walking.

Ah, so we did have the wrong girl – but at least we now knew who the right one was. Kim walked over to her. I called a quick 'Thank you' after the other girl and joined Kim.

'Hey,' Kim said.

'Hi,' Sandra replied. 'Is something wrong?'

'Not at all,' Kim said, glancing down at the mobile in Sandra's hands. She was in the process of writing a message to somebody. The mobile was a Blackberry.

'Can I borrow your phone for a moment?' Kim said.

'What? No you can't – you've got your own!' Sandra said, and pointed towards the personal radio clipped onto Kim's stab vest.

'Right, well, can you put it away in your pocket for a moment, then? There's something I need to talk to you about.'

I took a couple of strides away, and sat down on the steps. Kim was using her girl-talk voice and there wasn't much I could do by hovering but risk intimidating Sandra. I pretended to be incredibly bored and played with my iPhone, all the while keeping a close eye on both of them.

To my surprise, Sandra took Kim's suggestion, and put the phone in her trouser pocket, before leaning against the brick wall surrounding the courtyard of the estate. She folded her arms across her chest and glowered at my colleague.

'What?' she said.

'I hear there was a fight at school today,' Kim started.

'Yeah? So?'

'Well, the thing is, one of the girls who was in the fight got injured.'

'She's a bitch.'

'I can't really judge that; I don't know either of the girls. However, when there's a fight and somebody gets hurt, it's my job to find out what happened.'

'Did she call the cops? Fuck, that's so like her,' Sandra said, before realising she had sworn. 'Er, I mean . . . I didn't mean . . . I'm . . . Eh . . .' Sandra was looking so forlorn that Kim couldn't help but laugh.

'Don't worry,' she smiled, 'I won't arrest you for swearing. How's that?'

'You can do that?' Sandra said, wide-eyed. 'Arrest someone for swearing?'

'It depends. Are you going to swear some more?' Kim asked, and winked.

Sandra shook her head vigorously.

'I think we'll be fine then,' Kim said, and continued with the task in hand. 'Hey, Sandra, someone told us that you may have recorded the fight. On your mobile phone, maybe?'

From where I was sitting, I could see a change in Sandra. She tensed up, and one of her hands dropped down by her side, faux-casually. She had her hand resting over the pocket where her phone was.

'Is that bad?' she said. 'Is that illegal?'

'No, you can film whatever you want, whenever you want. Forget about that for now. Can I just talk to you about what happened?' Kim asked, whilst digging out her notebook.

Sandra nodded, and the two of them spent the next few minutes walking through what had happened: who said what and to whom, in what order, and why. Thankfully, Sandra proved to be a lot better at telling a coherent story than San had been.

Once Kim had outlined the whole story, and confirmed that Sandra had definitely filmed the incident, the time came to break the bad news.

'Well, I think that just about wraps it up, but now we have a bit of a problem – I'm going to have to borrow your phone for a while.'

'Why?'

'Well, you were witness to an assault, so we needed to take a statement from you, but what you have on your phone is evidence. I'm going to have to take your phone away to our lab, so our guys can take the video off your phone.'

'You can't do that!' Sandra said, loudly.

'Well, actually, I *can*.' Kim said. 'So, please, could I have your phone?'

'No. I use it all the time,' Sandra said. Kim glanced over at me and I shrugged. We had to take the phone.

'*DAAAAAAD!*' Sandra wailed.

A man sitting on one of the first-floor balconies peered over the railing at us.

'Uh. Hello, officers,' he stuttered, clearly confused to see two constables next to his daughter.

'What have you done now, Sandra?' he said, in the typical dad-joke fashion (delivered in the same tone as the hundreds of lines dads love to use whenever a police officer gets anywhere near them: 'He did it!' 'Oh no! They're coming to take me away', 'See, they're here because you didn't finish your sprouts last night.'

'They want to take my phone,' she shouted up.

'I'll be right down,' he called, and vanished towards the lifts. A fistful of seconds later, as the lift doors slid open, a tall man wearing a pair of glasses and a cigarette, along with well-worn flip-flops and a grim expression on his face, appeared.

'You can't take my daughter's phone,' he started immediately. 'She hasn't done anything wrong, has she?'

'Oh no, I didn't mean to give you that impression,' I hastily said. 'Your daughter is not under arrest, and she's not suspected of anything. The only thing is, she recorded an altercation on her mobile phone and we need to seize it as evidence.'

'That's bullshit,' he said.

'Dad! Language!' Sandra said hurriedly.

'Er, Yes. Sorry. But this isn't right. It's her phone, and you can't take it away from her,' the dad said. 'If you want the pictures, I'm sure Sandra would be happy to email them or put them on one of those USB-things for you. Wouldn't you, hon?'

Sandra nodded, her face brightening immediately; it looked as if she could keep her phone after all.

'Unfortunately, that's not going to be possible,' Kim said. 'In order for something to be useable as evidence, we need to take it off the device ourselves. In fact, it'll be our lab guys doing it. They'll do a statement about how they got the data off the phone and whether they believe it was tampered with or not. I'm not saying your daughter would do anything to the files, like accidentally erase them, edit them or anything like that, but it's simply the way we have to do things for something to stand up in court.'

My radio blipped into life.

'Two-zero receiving Mike Delta.'

I took a couple of steps away, without taking my eyes of the trio, and responded: 'Go ahead.'

'Are you guys nearly done over there? The late turn is coming on and they were just wondering when the car would be back.'

'Give us twenty minutes to wrap up. We'll be with you in half an hour,' I replied.

When I rejoined the conversation, there was a heated discussion going on.

'Give me the phone, Sandra,' the father said. Sandra produced the phone, and handed it over to her dad, who shoved it in the pocket of his cut-off jeans. 'You're not getting this phone. We bought it only a few months ago. Do you have any idea how expensive these damn things are?'

'Sir, I'm frightfully sorry, but don't worry,' Kim said. 'Your daughter will get her phone back, but we do need to seize it as evidence for now.'

'You can't just go around and take people's phones,' he said, shooting a long, lingering, angry stare at Kim.

'I completely understand that you are upset,' I interjected. 'But the truth is, we can most certainly take somebody's phone if we suspect that it contains evidence. Sandra said herself that the phone contains a video of a girl beating up another girl, and we will probably want to prosecute the assailant. To do that, we'll need the video evidence.'

My argument didn't seem to be working, so I decided to try another angle: 'How would you feel if Sandra had been assaulted, and you knew there was a video of the assault that could help get justice, but the person who filmed it didn't want to hand over their phone?'

'Yeah, well, you don't have the right,' the father said, feebly.

I could tell from the way he was looking at us that he did understand why we needed the video; he just didn't want to hand over the phone.

'I'm afraid I do. Under the Police and Criminal Evidence Act, section 19,' I said. 'There's another thing you have to keep in mind as well. If Sandra was to try and copy over the video files, but it turned out that they were corrupted for some reason, or they got deleted by accident, she would be under suspicion of tampering with evidence. That would be rather serious, wouldn't you think? Now, if our guys do something to delete the footage by accident, they'll have to write a statement about that and Sandra wouldn't be liable.'

'I understand all of that,' he said. 'So when could she get the phone back?'

'It shouldn't take too long,' I said, realising that I didn't actually know how long it was going to take. 'I don't know exactly how long, but I shouldn't think it would be more than a couple of weeks or so, at the most. After all, the phone itself wouldn't be evidence, just the video stored on there.'

'Can I call someone who knows the law, and find out?' he said.

'You can, but we're in a bit of a rush; we've been here for nearly an hour now, and the shift after us needs our car, so I'd like to be back in my car within five minutes,' I said.

Kim took a step forward: 'Sir, I really don't want to mention this, but if you don't hand the phone over voluntarily, we have the right to take it by force. I can see you're a reasonable guy, but I've explained everything to you and we really need to get going now.'

'Please,' she added, employing the mum-stare that few people can resist, 'the phone.'

Never in a million years did I think that little speech would work. Effectively threatening someone with violence rarely works, in my experience, but there's something very disarming about Kim. She was right, of course, we do have the legal right to take the phone by force, but actually explaining this to someone we were trying to convince was a bit of a gamble.

'Er,' the dad said, 'okay.'

He stuck his hand in his pocket and handed the phone over to Kim, who immediately turned to Sandra.

'Do you have a password on your Blackberry, in case the battery runs out?' she asked.

Sandra shook her head.

'Right,' Kim said, and pointed at an entry in her notebook. 'Now if you just sign here. This confirms that we've taken your phone and that you understand why.'

Sandra scribbled her signature at the bottom of the short entry in Kim's notebook.

'Thank you, Sandra,' she said. 'It's really important that people don't get away with bullying others like this, and your video is going to help make sure we can stop this from happening in the future. You've done a really good thing here today.'

We finished up with Sandra and her dad and left them on good terms. For sure, neither of them was happy that we'd taken the phone away, but both of them seemed to understand that we had to and that we had the right to do so.

When we'd climbed back into the car to go check the phone into evidence, I suddenly remembered an embarrassing episode from a few months ago, when I had seized a phone belonging to a drug dealer. 'Kim, did you remember to take the battery out of the phone?'

She shook her head, and immediately set about taking the phone apart to take the battery out. Blackberries are clever little devices – they can be wiped remotely, even if they are turned 'off' at the power key. There was probably little risk of Sandra doing that, to be fair, but you never knew.

When the time comes to copy the evidence off the phone, the forensic guys will hook it to a fresh battery, in a room that's completely shielded from radio signals, so that if anybody did try to wipe its memory, the signal wouldn't make it to the phone.

'Ha!' Kim said. 'Can you imagine if the phone got wiped after all that? We'd never hear the end of it . . .'

'Yeah, you ain't wrong,' I said. 'I'm just glad we didn't have to tussle with the dad. That could have gotten messy.'

She shot me a look: 'You need to get better at reading people. He was perfectly ready to hand over the phone; he just needed an excuse to do so, and I gave him one.'

I shrugged, and turned the BMW out of the estate, steeling myself for the hours of paperwork I still had to do after the day's shift, but still pleased I'd be off the streets before the evening fun started.

The stolen iPad

'Right,' the skipper said, as his eyes slid around the small assembly of plain-clothes officers in front of him. 'Jesus, you're a messy bunch.'

'If you were the fashion police,' he said to me and Simon, the only two in full uniform in the stuffy room, 'you'd have to arrest us all!'

We were on Operation Slate, an undercover job. Two female officers were to be placed, plain-clothed, in a busy bar that had become a hotspot for theft. The hope was that their tablet computer – an iPad – would be stolen, so we would be able to arrest the thieves right away.

Twenty minutes after the briefing, we had installed ourselves in and outside the bar we were covering.

Though we were all in close vicinity, we would communicate by radio alone. I went on the *Event 2* channel that was reserved for our sting operation. Simon stayed on the normal despatch channel on the radio, to keep half an ear on things going on around the rest of the borough.

'Radio check from uniformed units on Operation Slate,' I radioed in.

'CCTV receiving,' one of the team members in the bar's CCTV room radioed back.

'Safety receiving,' the team guarding Lisa and Miranda – our officers with the iPad – added.

'Spotter Alpha receiving,' said another officer who was charged with just milling around the nightclub looking for known suspects and keeping an eye on things.

Then my radio beeped twice. One of the undercover officers had a radio in their purse, with a pair of buttons on the inside of the bag. One of the buttons sends a beep; the other sends an urgent assistance signal. Two beeps meant 'okay', so I guess they were receiving us.

We are involved in operations like this every few weeks, targeting whatever crime hotspots we have around the borough. We usually target different types of theft, including bicycle theft, pick-pocketing, shoplifting, among others, usually guided by the areas where the SMT[63] in the borough feels our statistics are weakest.

The jobs tend to be either incredibly busy or completely dead. So far, this was the latter. Simon and I were strolling up and down the street outside the nightclub, with my radio silent apart from the occasional radio check.

The streets around the club quarter were relatively well patrolled; six officers were doing big loops around the bar district, and every 20 minutes or so, I'd have a chance for a quick chat to catch up on some of the gossip. It's a perk of these operations; you're working with people that aren't on the same team as you, so you get a chance to catch up and have a natter with officers you don't know as well, or haven't seen in a while.

At one in the morning, about three hours into the operation, my radio woke up from its slumber.

'All teams stand by; we have some suspicious activity near the girls.'

'Standing by,' the safety team replied.

---

[63] Senior Management Team

I whistled to Simon, who was giving incredibly detailed directions to two attractive blondes in high heels. He waved back, said his fond farewell and started walking towards the club on his side of the street.

'It's an IC1 male, around five foot tall, blue striped shirt, carrying a small backpack over one shoulder,' the CCTV team transmitted. 'He is sitting down, looking around. He is at the end of the cubicle with the bag holding our package. Don't look at him.'

Inside the club, there were six officers who desperately wanted to get a closer look at their suspect, but forced themselves to stare at each other instead.

'Our view is blocked,' the CCTV operator said. 'No visual.'

'I see him,' one of the safety officers radioed back, barely legible over the music in the background.

Simon and I were on opposite sides of the door to the nightclub; if the thief did steal the iPad, he would probably try to make a quick exit, and then it would be our turn to leap into action. Simon was leaning against a barrier where about 20 people were waiting to be let into the club.

My radio suddenly spat out a 15-second burst of loud club music, but no recognisable words.

'Safety, are you okay?' the CCTV team transmitted, followed by a long burst of silence, during which my full concentration was on the earpiece I was wearing.

'Safety, confirm status. Spotters, go check on them,' the CCTV team transmitted, after what seemed like an absolute eternity.

I was waiting for my radio to give a meaningful response, when I heard a commotion on the far side of the club doors. Simon had turned around, and was shouting at a young man.

'Mate, shut up and listen,' he shouted. 'If this gentleman says you have had enough to drink, then that's his prerogative. Go home.'

I sighed; it's a scene we see a dozen times on any given Friday or Saturday night; a group of young lads had been ejected from one club for being a drunken gaggle of nuisance-makers and were trying to sneak into the next club. The bouncers use their own radios to warn each other about the worst grief-magnets, and so when the inebriated good-for-noughts are ejected from one club, chances are they won't be doing any more drinking that night. It's a pretty good system, particularly because it's a lot easier to deal with troublemakers outside a club than inside one.

The group of youths was six strong, and they were obviously disinclined to listen to Simon. I glanced at the door for a second, then reached for my radio, changed the channel to despatch and quickly transmitted.

'Mike Delta receiving five-nine-two.'

'Five-nine-two, go ahead.'

'We're on Operation Slate. I'm outside the Summer Fiesta nightclub, and could do with some additional help to clear away a group of six inebriated males.'

'Received,' the operator replied, and then proceeded to transmit a request for some extra backup.

I switched back to the operation channel and caught the tail end of a transmission.

'. . . the door.'

'I was on another channel,' I said. 'Update, please?'

'Coming, Matt! Yellow shirt!' one of the safety officers shouted down the radio. I whirled around, and spotted a man with a yellow shirt dart out of the club, clutching Lisa's bag. He didn't even pause long enough to spot me in my uniform; he simply ran straight past me.

'Shit,' I transmitted. 'Get some guys out here, I can't leave Simon by himself,' I said, my eyes on the man who was sprinting down the road. The argument between Simon and the young men was escalating.

About 30 seconds later, several of the spotters and the two safety officers came bursting out through the doors.

'What the fuck?' one of them shouted. 'All you had to do was to stop the little bastard!'

I waved him off, and turned my attention to Simon, who was now physically intervening between the 'ingress/egress security advisor' (that's a bouncer to you and me) and two of the lads who were causing trouble. I walked over and got involved, and half a second later the three spotters joined us.

'Stand back,' one of them called. 'Police!'

The group of youths was momentarily confused. The plain-clothes officers had hauled warrant cards attached to lanyards out of their pockets and donned them around their necks to identify them as police, but at the same time, two additional security guys had shown up; they were also wearing their IDs around their necks.

'Fuck you, you ain't police,' one of the youngsters said to the bouncers, as one of his friends was dragging at his arm.

'Dude, they're totally police, let's get out of here,' he said.

Slowly, the guys gathered their wits. Just when they had decided to go, a van containing half a dozen uniformed units arrived. The drunk boys seemed to sober up rather impressively quickly at the sight of them, and executed their previously made plan of making a hasty disappearance. They started running down the road. We let them go; they had been loud and obnoxious, and perhaps shoved Simon around a little bit, but nothing they'd get prosecuted for. Besides, we had bigger fish to fry.

I turned around. The whole operation team had come out of the nightclub.

'Why didn't you stop him, Delito?' Seventy-one's voice boomed.

'Er . . . Simon . . .' I stuttered.

Sergeant Thomas, who had been leading the operation, piped up.

'Not to worry, lads,' he said, and fished an iPhone out of his pocket. 'I can track the iPad with this thing.'

Apple's Find My iPhone/iPod/iPad feature is great, but it's not perfect – it's useful for finding out where your iPhone is at any given time, but if it gets stolen and ends up in a council estate somewhere – as stolen things are often wont to do – you've got a problem: we can tell which building the device is in, but there could be dozens, if not hundreds, of flats stacked on top of each other, and we wouldn't be able to bust in through every single door looking for one device.

'What does this mean?' the skipper said, pointing non-specifically at the iPhone's screen.

'Can I?' I asked. I'm a bit of an Apple fanboy, and I've used the system before.

'It says it can't find the iPad,' I said, after pressing various options on his iPhone screen for a while.

'Damn,' the sarge said. 'He must have disconnected from the WiFi.'

'Umm . . . What do you mean?' I asked.

'Well, if he disconnects from the WiFi, we can't find him until he connects to a different WiFi.'

'You've got to be kidding me,' I said. 'Is it not a 3G iPad?'

The sergeant stared at me blankly.

'What . . .' he said, 'do you mean?'

'You bought the iPad thing especially for these operations, right?' I said to the boss of the Clubs and Vice team.

'Yeah.'

'So, er, which iPad did you buy?'

'Don't be an idiot, Delito,' he said. 'This is the Metropolitan

Police. You shouldn't have to ask; I bought the cheapest one, of course.'

'Oh, Jesus,' I said, rubbing my forehead with my fingertips.

'What?' demanded Simon.

'The top-model iPads have 3G and GPS built in. Like on a phone. So, if we'd bought one of those, the iPad would know exactly where it was, and it would have an Internet connection anywhere there is mobile phone coverage,' I explained. 'But instead, we bought the cheapest version, which only has WiFi, and no GPS. The one we bought never knows exactly where it is, it can only guess its location based on what WiFi networks it can see . . . And it only has a network when it is connected to WiFi.'

Nine pairs of eyes stared at me blankly.

'Fer feck's sake,' I said. 'Do I really have to spell it out? Basically, we won't have any idea where that iPad is until our thief connects it to a WiFi network. Which, if he has any sense, he won't do. If he formats the damn thing, we're royally fucked; we won't get our iPad back, and the guy will get away with it.'

'But . . . I have Find My iPad right here,' Sergeant Thomas said, wiggling his iPhone in the air desperately. 'Bollocks,' he concluded, wisely.

The sarge stood still for a second, weighing his options. Then he started ordering people around: 'Okay, Delito, you know about this geek stuff. Simon, stick with me, and Tracy, you come with us as well. The rest of you, you're dismissed. Write up a quick MG11[64] about the theft, and email it to me before you head home.'

'Let's see if we can't find our iPad,' he added grimly to those of us who had been 'lucky' enough to be chosen to stay behind.

'Bollocks to that,' Tracy said. 'I need a cuppa.'

The sergeant sighed.

---

[64] Witness statement

'Yeah, me too. Let's go,' he said, and led the way to one of the late-night coffee bars that had recently popped up in the area. The coffee bars were apparently opened especially to cater to stoned hipsters, hip stoners – and us.

As we leaned over our steaming cups of coffee, the sarge prodded his iPhone whilst the rest of us looked beaten.

'Do you know what the kid looks like?' Simon asked, half-heartedly.

'Yes, but we were tracking the wrong guy on the CCTV for most of the evening. We had the fella in the striped shirt, he was looking well dodgy, but after the other guy ran off with the iPad we finally took him aside and it turned out he was just pilled off his face,' Sergeant Thomas said, shaking his head. 'We did catch the little bastard on one of the cameras, though. I emailed a copy of the image to my phone, hang on . . .'

After a couple of minutes' worth of fiddling – about a minute and 57 seconds longer than it ought to have taken – Sergeant Thomas held up his phone.

'Never seen 'im before,' Simon said, after poring over the shot for a moment. The rest of us repeated similar sentiments.

We spent another ten minutes in the café finishing our coffee. Just before we got up to leave, Thomas had another look at his iPhone.

'I've got him!' he said.

Simon and I leapt up and slid around the table to look over the sergeant's shoulder.

Tracy, who was sitting next to the sarge had a clear view: 'He's just off the borough,' he said, 'but only about ten minutes away. Have we got a car?'

'Er . . .' the skipper replied, tentatively. 'Technically, no. We sent them all on their way home. I figured we could catch a lift later.'

'Any units near the Coffee Bucket?' I threw myself on my radio.

Tracy walked to the counter to pay for our coffees, whilst Simon and Sergeant Thomas kept their eyes on the little iPad icon in the middle of the map display.

'Unit calling for backup near Coffee Bucket; Mike Delta two-eight receiving.'

'Two-eight, cancel, cancel, we don't need backup. We just need a lift. Do you have ten minutes?'

'Yeah, of course,' came the reply. 'On the hurry-up?' he asked.

'Yes, yes.'

'Aaaalrighty then,' the driver said, and halfway through his atrocious Jim Carrey impression, we heard the sirens of a caged van whine into life over the radio. 'For you? Special price. Get me a brew, will ya?'

Tracy overheard the conversation via his radio, turned around and retraced his steps back to the counter to order a cup of tea for the van driver.

Moments later, sirens came to a halt outside the coffee shop, and we all poured out and climbed into the van.

'Hey, Joe,' I said, recognising the driver and passing him his tea.

'Thank you for your expedience,' Thomas said. 'Step on it, we need to get to Garyson Rise double-quick.'

He flashed his iPhone at Joe to show where we were going.

'Aye, boss,' Joe said. He placed his drink in the cup holder and pulled away. Laughing, he added, 'Are you going to the Starbucks up there? I thought you guys just *had* a coffee'.

Tracy and I looked at each other. Garyson Rise is just outside our borough, in an area where there isn't usually a lot of trouble, so I'm not very familiar with it.

'Seriously? There's a Starbucks?' I asked. 'What else is there?'

'Oh, not much, really,' Joe said. 'Couple of pizza joints. Delivery places, mostly. One of those Internet places and a Tesco, but I think it closes at midnight,' he rambled on.

'Screw the Starbucks,' I said.

'Take us to the Internet place,' Tracy added, finishing my thought.

'But kill the sirens and lights before we get there,' Simon said completing our train of thought.

Finally, for the first time all night, we were working as a team.

As we came up to Garyson Rise, Joe cut the sirens. He left the blues on as we pulled through a red light. Then he shut the flashers off as well, and stopped in a bus stop a few doors down from the Internet shop. The shutters covering the windows were down, but the door shutter was open and there was a dim ray of light spilling out onto the pavement.

'I'll go in. You guys stop him from getting away again,' Tracy said.

Simon and Tracy got out of the van and Tracy took up position next to the shop.

'Fuck me, where did you learn to drive, Joe?' I said, keeping my eyes on the shop front. Joe mumbled something about hiring a limo instead, if I didn't like his driving. The sergeant and I climbed out of the van and approached the door from the other side.

Once we were in position, Tracy nodded to Simon, before turning back and nodding to me. We were ready . . . He quickly checked to make sure none of his police paraphernalia was showing, before he casually strolled into the Internet shop, his police radio on mute in his back pocket. Tracy's undercover stab vest and other equipment in a covert vest were hidden under his oversized zippered hoodie.

He came walking out again after a minute, sipping a can of Coke. He didn't look at any of us, until he was out of the dull light-cone from the door. When he was out of sight, he looked over his shoulder to see if he'd been followed, before quickly unzipping his hoodie and shooting some instructions over to Simon. A second later, Simon's voice came over the radio.

'There are two guys in there, and they're using an iPad. Tracy says it doesn't have that hideous pink cover on it, but it looks like they have a fair amount of second-hand stuff for sale behind the counter. It could be anywhere. One of the men is our man from the bar,' Simon said.

Tracy grabbed the radio from Simon, ignoring the one he had sticking out of his back pocket.

'I recognise the other guy, too; he's a nasty piece of work. I don't think he clocked me, but I nicked him for running a prostitution racket a few year years back. Turkish bloke, in a blue shirt. He put up quite a fight last time I nicked him, so be careful.'

'Should we go in now or wait?' the skipper asked.

'Now. Let's get the little fucker,' Tracy said.

'Let's do it,' the skipper said, reaching for his torch. I did the same, and saw Simon producing a torch as well.

Simon was first in though the door.

'Police, don't move,' he shouted, and pointed his torch straight in the face of the guy with the yellow shirt.

I aimed my torch into the eyes of the second man, who was seated behind the table, but he dropped the iPad in front of him, leapt to his feet and dived out of sight to the left of us. Tracy leapt forward and grabbed hold of our yellow-shirted scoundrel, and within seconds he had his prisoner bent over the table with a set of handcuffs keeping his arms behind his back.

Simon and I edged forward, trying to locate the man in blue over the racket being caused by Tracy trying to search his prisoner and Sergeant Thomas radioing in a status report. The man seemed to have vanished into thin air. I stuck my head carefully around the corner and spotted a stairway going down into darkness.

'He's gone down the stairs,' I called. I turned around to see whether Simon was still following me, and caught a face-full of his ludicrously bright LED torch, which caused me to lose whatever night vision I might have had up to that point.

'Sorry, mate,' he mumbled.

'Let's see if we can find him,' I said, and started descending the stairs, my torch piercing the darkness. I heard a clicking sound next to my head; it was Simon, trying a light switch. Nothing.

We continued down the creaking stair. At the bottom, there was a small, narrow hallway going left and right. We stopped and listened, and I took a step to the right, letting Simon step off the stairs with a step to the left. We couldn't hear anything.

Simon swung his torch around, and took a couple of steps down the corridor.

Suddenly, I heard an almighty crash and a shout.

'Whattafuuuuuuuuuu—' Simon wailed, as his torch went spinning away into the dark corridor, creating a ghoulish shadow play on the walls as the light from his torch picked up all sorts of rubbish on the floor.

'Aaaaaaaaaah,' Simon shouted again. In the light of my own torch, I could see him grabbing his arm. I also spotted his assailant; it was the Turkish man Tracy had warned us about before we entered the shop.

I reached up to my radio and pressed the orange button next to my antenna.

'Urgent assistance required,' I shouted. 'Basement of the Internet shop, 33 Garyson Rise, we're under attack from a man with a stick.'

I paused briefly to think whether there's anything else I needed to say: 'Get us an ambulance as well, Mike Delta two-eight-eight got whacked.'

With that, I turned my torch off.

There are few things police officers care about more than their torches. You'll inevitably lose your torch eventually, but that doesn't stop me from investing some serious cash into a top-quality light source; I use the thing nearly every night shift, so it makes sense to get a proper one. Some officers choose to use Maglite-style torches so they can double as nightsticks, but I don't quite see the point. I already have a police-issue Asp – or a gravity friction-lock baton, as it's officially called – which is manufactured specifically for slapping people about, so I have no idea why anyone would choose to carry a heavy flashlight. My torch is a Night-Ops Gladius, a tactical flashlight that was apparently made for mounting on an assault rifle or a pistol. Since the Met hasn't deigned to provide me with one of these lead-redistribution devices, I use the torch on its own. I chose it for several reasons: it's as solid as can be; it's the right size to be used as a Kubotan (a small hand-to-hand combat weapon); and, most importantly, it has a rapid strobe mode, a feature that has saved my bacon more than once.

With a quick twist of the torch's rear cap, you can prepare the strobe mode. Next, point it at someone's eyes and press the back of the cap to activate it. If you're at the receiving end of that treatment, it's extremely disorienting; the only thing you'll see is the strobing of the light – the person behind the light becomes completely invisible.

This seemed a perfect occasion to exploit my torch's functionality. I flicked my Gladius into the strobe mode, passed it into my left hand, and drew and racked my Asp with my right.

I could just make out the man from the light of Simon's torch, which had come to rest pointing at the wall behind him. He was hiding next to the half-opened door, as Simon lay yelping on the floor, pushing himself towards me with his legs.

'You okay?' I asked him, knowing the answer.

'Do I fucking sound all right?' he barked. 'He twatted me in the fucking arm, didn't he?'

'Hey! You!' I called out to the man. 'You saw us, you know we've got two more officers upstairs, and we've got a vanload more coppers coming. Put down the bat, you can't win.'

An unprintable malediction ruptured from behind the door.

'I'll give you five seconds,' I said. 'Then I'm coming for you.'

I could see him take a firmer grip of his aluminium bat as he tensed in anticipation; I also heard a faint creaking on the stairs next to me. They must have finished loading our other prisoner into the back of the van, because both Tracy and Sergeant Thomas were on the stairs, batons drawn, ready to spring into action.

'Five . . .' I said. Simon staggered to his feet next to the stairs, and leant against the walls.

'Four . . .' I called a few seconds later. I whispered to Simon, 'Take my torch. When I say One, lean as far forward as you can.'

'Three . . .' I said out loud, before dropping my voice to a whisper again '. . . and hold the button on the back pressed in. Whatever happens, keep it aimed at his eyes.'

'Two . . .' I called out to the man. Then slid my torch into the hand of Simon's uninjured arm, double-checking he had a firm grip of the torch before I let go of his hand.

'Got that?' I whispered.

'ONE!' I called, and dropped to the floor with all the grace and finesse of a narcoleptic cow.

Simon shouted a battle cry that would make a banshee sob with envy, as he pressed the button on the back of the torch. The super-bright LED bulb started strobing rapidly, catching the man square in the face. I crawled as fast as I could, on all fours like a dog, along the floor.

With the first few strobes, I could see his wide-open eyes. The next few flashes illuminated his whole face as he moved out of his hiding place, taking a firmer grip of his bat and trying to shrink away from the bright light being beamed at him.

I could see the expression on his face change with each pulse of light.

It showed his gritted teeth.

It showed a face that was making the decision to fight for his life.

He raised his bat. But then, suddenly, realised something was wrong; the source of the strobing light and manic cry wasn't coming closer.

Just as the penny dropped, my baton connected with the side of his left shin. The man screamed and I didn't waste any time. I leapt to a position behind him. He was holding his bat with his right hand, as his left went down to his shin. I whirled around and put my whole weight behind my baton, aiming for the side of his upper arm. To the sound of a nausea-inducing snap, the baton thumped into his arm less than a second after it had reduced the nerves in his lower leg to a concerto of agony. From the 'snap', I was pretty certain I had broken his arm.

I grabbed my cuffs out of their holder, but before I was able to get close enough to apply them to the now-squealing man, another set of hands reached out of the dark, grabbed him and hauled him to the ground, pressing his face against the dusty floor. Tracy's torch clicked on and suddenly the whole messy scene was well lit.

He wasn't one for wasting time; Simon's attacker was in handcuffs before he had time to take another breath.

By now I was sitting on the floor, my back to a wall, panting. As the adrenaline of our sneak attack wore off, I could feel my knees hurting. I looked down to see I was bleeding from my right knee; my left one was badly scraped as well but somehow wasn't leaking, though the trouser legs on both legs were torn.

'Extra points for creativity,' Simon said drily, and limped his way up the stairs, muttering something about ambulances.

One of those shifts

'We've had a report of a burglary in progress at the MumToBe on 53 Lower Street,' the call came over the radio. 'Graded I, Graded India.'

I leapt up and grabbed the coffee from the table in front of me. I must have squeezed a little bit too enthusiastically on the Styrofoam cup.

The lid popped off.

The cup buckled.

It slid from between my fingers.

The cup hit the table, sending a fountain of steaming hot coffee straight up towards me. I saw it coming in slow-mo, but thanks to a bona-fide miracle, it failed to hit me in the face. Instead, it cascaded down the front of my Metvest and into my lap.

I swore and then, leaving the enormous puddle of coffee where it was, grabbed some napkins, and furiously rubbed my crotch with them, as I sped out of the cafeteria, transmitting at the same time.

'Show two-four,' I said.

'Last transmitting, what's your shoulder number please?'

'It's PC five-nine-two Mike Delta, Matt Delito.'

'Received. We'll send the CAD to your MDT,' they concluded,

and proceeded to send the notes for the current call to the mobile data terminal built into my police car.

'Received, thanks,' I said, and climbed into the vehicle.

The fabric our uniform trousers are made of is truly, profoundly horrible: scratchy and static and not particularly comfortable. Though, it does have two advantages: it dries very quickly and, being dark blue, stains don't show up that easily.

However, as I sped out of the gate, blue strobes reflecting on the walls around me, the formerly scalding-hot coffee was cooling down rapidly, and a chill ran up my spine. I glanced down: there was a hugely visible wet patch on the front of my trousers.

In moments, I turned the car down Lower Street, and arrived at the MumToBe shop front.

'Show two-four on location,' I transmitted, as I brought the car to a very rapid halt. I got out, grabbed my torch and peered into the shop for a closer look.

The scene was dead.

'I can't see any sign of the burglars, but the glass in the entry door has been smashed in,' I transmitted, realising grimly what that would mean.

There was only one thing for it. I couldn't do a drive-around looking for the suspects. Nobody was in the shop to look after it, and with the front door completely smashed in, I couldn't leave it unguarded.

As soon as we arrive on scene, it becomes our responsibility that nothing further is stolen, so I wouldn't be able to leave until the door had been boarded up or the owners of the store had returned to look after their wares.

I got back on the radio, on the spare channel.

'I'm going to need someone who can board up a shop door,' I transmitted.

There was a moment's pause before the response came: 'Ah, I may have some bad news for you.'

'What do you mean?'

'Well, there was some unrest in one of the neighbouring boroughs earlier today, and there seems to be quite a long wait before anybody will be able to come out and board up a shop front.'

'Er. Could you give me an estimate?'

'I could, but you're not going to like it.'

'Go on?'

'Eight.'

'What? in the morning?' I asked, looking at my watch. It had only just turned 10 p.m.

'Sorry, buddy. We'll try to send someone to relieve you as soon as we can, but for now, hang tight!'

I looked up and down the street. The whole stretch of road, as far as I could see, was completely deserted. Not a single open shop, not one pedestrian. Even the lamp-posts seemed to spill their light on the road only with great reluctance. *Great.* I'd be spending the next few hours guarding a ghost town.

I grabbed some POLICE LINE DO NOT CROSS cordon tape from the back of the Panda, and cordoned off the area in front of the shop, from the corner of the shutters, via a lamp-post, to the next set of shutters along.

After that, there was nothing to do but wait.

I settled in, standing against the wall.

The first 20 minutes were a bit slow.

The next 20 minutes were dreadfully boring.

The next 20 minutes were deathly boring.

In the 20 minutes after that, I started to lose my will to live. To make matters worse, I discovered that I really, really needed to go to the bathroom.

My watch beeped. It was 11 p.m. My radio was beginning its slow-building crescendo in the Friday-night symphony of destruction: there was a relatively serious accident where a bus driver had run down a pedestrian; there were three separate armed robberies, which appeared to be linked, and the robbery squad, on motorbikes, had support from four additional motorbikes from Traffic, trying to chase down the moped-riding robbers. There was a huge fight among several groups of travellers, which seemed to spread slowly from pub to pub somewhere in the south of the borough; there was a sudden death of a woman in her mid-30s that was considered suspicious. Later, another traffic collision was added to the mix, this time between a car and two bicyclists, one of whom had tragically expired on the scene already.

If that sounds busy, it wasn't the half of it: a report had been called in of a man shouting threats to kill at a group of teenagers. The man had been spotted with what appeared to be a shotgun, and the helicopter and several Trojan units were called in. The main dispatch channel was taken over by a shooting incident, and the working channel was changed to another channel. The earlier brawl slowly got even more out of hand, and fighting had now been reported at four different pubs. CS gas was deployed in two of the locations, and the Territorial Support Group was called in to try and deal with the fighting, which was now technically three riots and an affray.

And all the while, I was standing outside the Mum To Be, with a wet and cold crotch, and a desperate need to go for a wee, powerlessly listening as my teammates were being pushed to hell and back.

Then, finally, my radio said something actually directed at me.

'Five-nine-two receiving Mike Delta?' the radio said.

'Yes! Receiving!' I said, elated that I might finally be relieved.

'You still on your last?'

'Yes, yes.'

'How long do you think you're going to be?'

'Er . . . You tell me? I'm waiting for someone to come board up this shop.'

'Oh. Right,' the CAD operator said. 'The next shift are going to need your car. We'll send someone to come pick it up, and see about getting you relieved.'

'Received,' I said drily.

A few minutes later, a car showed up with two officers. One of them left right away in the car they had come in, heading off to help out with the brawl, but I managed to convince the other to stand watch for a few minutes whilst I walked to the McDonald's around the corner to use the bathroom and buy some water.

'You didn't make it, then,' he said when I returned.

'Huh?'

'Looks like you've pissed yourself, mate,' he laughed.

I looked down.

Oh yes.

The coffee stain was significantly more visible than I'd hoped it would be.

'It's coffee,' I said, but there was nobody listening; he had already vanished down the road in my car, leaving me with only the smell of burning rubber and the echoes of his sirens for company.

The echoes died out.

'Thanks a lot, guys,' I said to myself.

I was outside the shop for another hour and a half before an officer arrived on foot.

'Hey!' he said brightly.

'Hi,' I replied.

'What are you doing here, then?' he asked

'Er . . . Waiting for you, I hope?'

'I dunno, are you? I'm just wandering around on foot patrol at the moment,' he said.

Angry, I grabbed my radio.

'Mike Delta receiving five-nine-two?'

'Go ahead?'

'I was just wondering if you guys would be able to arrange for me to be relieved?'

'Er . . . I don't have you as active on my system,' the CAD op said.

'I assure you I'm most certainly active. And I've been on this crime scene for nearly four hours,' I snapped.

'Stand by,' the operator replied, and continued, 'Mike Delta receiving two-eight-one.'

The officer standing next to me looked down at his radio, and reached for his transmit button.

'Receiving,' he said.

'Are you free to deal?'

'Yes, yes.'

'You are on foot, correct? In the Lower Street area?'

'Yes, yes.'

'Could you make your way to the MumToBe on Lower Street?'

'Yes, yes.'

'There's an officer there who needs to be relieved.'

'Yes, yes.'

'Mike Delta five-nine-two receiving?' the operator continued, addressing me this time.

'Yes, yes,' I replied, mirroring my colleague wearily.

'Your relief is on its way.'

'Yes, yes.'

'Two-eight is on their way back to the station with a prisoner,' they said, referring to the call sign of the caged van. 'I'll get them to pick you up on the way.'

'Yes, yes.'

I stood around, chatting with two-eight-one for a few minutes.

'Need a drink?' I asked the officer.

'Yeah, if you wouldn't mind?'

I walked to the McDonald's again to get my relief a cup of coffee and a large water. When I returned, the van was there, waiting for me, finally.

It had been an absolute killer of a shift, and I had missed out on all of it, protecting a broken window pane from curious cats and inquisitive foxes for more than half of my shift. Frankly, all I wanted to do was go home, bury my face in a pillow and sleep for 12 hours.

As I got in the van, two-eight-one called after me: 'Hey, Delito,' he shouted.

I turned around.

'It looks like you pissed yourself,' he said, and waved a goodbye.

'Thanks, I know,' I called back, and slumped back in the van, on my way back to the police station.

The arrest enquiry

'Delito,' the skipper snapped, peering over his stack of loosely arranged papers.

I looked up.

'What are you, six years old?'

'What? I . . . I didn't even do anything,' I stuttered, but the sergeant's eyes confirmed that my half-hearted lie was never going to be believed.

I bowed my head and mumbled a 'Sorry, sarge', which was greeted by a cacophony of laughter from the rest of my team.

We had been carrying out a series of practical pranks on each other all week, and I'd managed to be the first person to get caught out, mid-prank.

I spent the next few minutes fiddling with my handcuff keys, trying to release the cuff that was linking Pete's arm to the radiator – and just in time, too. The inspector walked into the briefing room, and we all leapt to our feet. Pete hid the fact that he still had a cuff attached to his arm by placing his hand behind his back.

Some inspectors really like to, er, inspect, but thankfully the unfortunately named Inspector Michael Hunt (he insists, for obvious reasons, on being called 'Michael') has a slightly more relaxed take on things.

Inspector Hunt counted the number of faces, before waving us back down into our seats.

'Nice one, Delito,' Pete whispered to me. 'I didn't see that one coming. Of course, I'll get my revenge – you'd better keep a cuff key handy . . .' he said, grinning.

It was one of those unexpectedly hot days that sometimes arrive even before the beginning of spring. The kind of day you remember from childhood, when you'd sneak outside without a jacket for the first time in the year, without any real risk of your mum shouting at you for it.

'Pretty light shift today,' the inspector grunted at our shift sergeant.

'Yeah. Couple of people on training, four are in court to testify on that bar brawl back in November, one's off ill, and a small group are on secondment to CO eleven[65], some sort of training ahead of the Olympics, I think,' he replied.

'Righty-oh,' the inspector said, looking around the room. 'There's still almost a dozen of you, so let's wrap up this briefing and go hunting.'

We were given our postings as usual, but for reasons unknown to me, I was put on caged-van duty. It's not a bad posting, really, but it had been a long time since I'd been in anything but a Panda or the area car.

'Five-nine-two and two-two-three,' the skipper said, looking over at Pete and myself. 'Before we get too many bodies in, could the two of you go and deal with an arrest inquiry? Take seven-two-three with you.'

Once we'd left the briefing room, I walked over to the Borough Intelligence Unit based at our station and asked them to print us off a copy of the arrest inquiry we were meant to go to.

[65] The Metropolitan Police public order branch

'I've already got the CAD,' I said as I returned to my team, and triumphantly held up the six sheets of A4 paper, still warm from the printer. 'Who wants coffee?'

We all piled into the mess at the police station. I ordered a round of coffees (the ground stuff that we have to pay for, not the pitiful slop that comes out of the free machine), and Pete skim-read the CAD printout to see what we were up for.

'Right,' Pete said. 'Looks like we're looking for a, um, Stephanie Eng . . . Engu . . .'

'You what?' I said. 'I'm sure it was some dude we were looking for?'

'It says "Stephanie",' Pete said. 'Oh, wait . . .'

I grabbed the papers from him.

'You plum . . . It says Stéphane. That's like Steven. And the last name is Nguimgo,' I said, hoping I hadn't butchered the guy's last name too badly.

I continued to scan the report.

'He's from Cameroon . . . Wanted for serious assault at work . . . He works in a warehouse . . . Wow . . .' – I paused – 'Says here he smacked first his boss, then a co-worker, with a crowbar – all over an argument about some food in the break-room fridge. Lovely fellow.'

'Remind me why they aren't sending the BSU to deal with this guy,' seven-two-three, affectionately known as Bernard, or Bernard Bernard, piped up; it was the first thing he had said all day. 'Sounds like he's a piece of work, and at least those meatheads are padded,' Bernard concluded, before glancing over to Pete, who takes any secondments to the Borough Support Unit that are on offer. 'No offence, of course.'

'None taken,' Pete answered. However, his face said otherwise. Bernard and Pete had had a falling out over something or other. Again. They are both great police officers, but they are simultaneously too similar *and* too different to play nicely together.

'Anyway, last known address is here, where they send his pay-slips,' I said, pointing at the address. 'So I guess we go take a look there. It's only a ten-minute drive.'

Turning to Bernard I asked, 'You want a lift with us, or are you taking a separate car?'

Bernard decided to grab a Panda and make his way separately. Not a bad idea: when you're on caged-van duty, you can be called away from less urgent tasks, and it's a pain in the arse if you're stuck on the van as a passenger when that happens.

Thirty minutes later, we were outside a block of flats in a particularly grim ex-council estate, discussing amongst ourselves how best to get into the building. We could have rung the doorbell, of course, but when you're going to places on official duty – especially if you're going on an arrest enquiry – it makes sense to not announce your presence until you're ready to do so.

'Anyone got a fireman's key?' Pete asked.

'I do,' I answered, and started rooting around in my Metvest for the short length of metal that opens nearly all estate outer doors when inserted into the hole marked 'fire' (normally up high, above the buzzers or door entry system), but it had gone missing.

'Gis here, then,' Pete said.

'Someone's nicked it,' I concluded. My key *had* been clipped to the left pocket of my Metvest with a carabineer, but it was no longer there. I suddenly remembered that I had left my Metvest hanging outside my locker at the police station a few days before. I had been dealing with a grim traffic accident, and in an effort to try and clean off the blood, I had managed to convince the drycleaners around the corner to clean my vest for me. When I got it back, it was still a bit damp, so I had left it out to dry out properly. Someone must have taken my fireman's key then.

'Fuck's sake,' Pete said, before walking back to the Panda, rummaging around in the bag he keeps in the boot of the police car and returning with his own key. We were inside in no time.

It turned out the elevator was broken, so we had to take the stairs. On the way up, I was moaning about my missing fireman's key.

'That was the third bloody key I've lost,' I said.

'You should have learned then, shouldn't you?' Pete said. 'Nothing's safe in a police station.'

He's right. The amount of stuff that goes missing at police stations is absolutely mind-boggling. Pieces of uniform are particularly prone to sprout legs and go walkies. Nobody ever gets caught nicking each other's stuff, either. It's bizarre.

Just as I was coming to the climax of my rant – 'How can people get away with nicking stuff in the building with the highest per-square-feet number of police officers in London!' – we arrived at the fourth-floor flat.

I'm not a huge fan of this estate. It's particularly out of the way, neither our patrol cars nor those of the borough south of ours tend to be in the area. If you need assistance, it's not easy. On this particular occasion, I concluded we'd be fine. There were three of us: Pete is built like a brick outhouse; Bernard does some sort of martial art ('I'm all Martial, no Art,' he likes to say – I think the martial art in question is *Krav Maga*, but I'm not sure); and I'm pretty useful when the proverbial push comes to shove, as well.

Pete took the lead, and rapped on the door with his knuckles. Meanwhile, I bent down and took a peek through the letterbox. I spotted someone dressed in a towel move from the hallway into a room to the left-hand side.

'Police!' I shouted into the letterbox. 'Open up!'

Nothing.

'Police!' I tried again. 'I've seen you! If you don't come open the door right now, we'll find our own way in!'

There was no sound from inside the flat.

'Do these flats have rear entrances?' I asked the others.

'Not that I know of. There may be a window going out the side, but I don't think there's a roof or anything they can climb onto,' Bernard replied.

'Well then . . .' I said to them, before shouting through the letterbox one last time, banging on the door with the butt of my baton, 'If you do not open up right now, we'll have to open it for you.'

'Do you need this door open, boss?' Pete asked.

'Yeah, I just said, didn't I? . . . But, we should probably go get the Big Red Key.'

The Big Red Key is what we call the battering ram that's bolted down behind the driver's seat in the caged van.

'Fuck *that* for a sack of cow's testicles,' Pete said colourfully (if slightly zoologically inaccurately). 'The lift's broken, isn't it?'

He took a step back, and gave the door an almighty kick. It creaked, but stubbornly resisted the attack. Pete kicked again, and this time the door flew open. In the blow, the top hinge had become loose as well, so as the door flew inwards, it swayed back and forth briefly, before the screws came loose from the rotten wood at the bottom and the whole door went tumbling inwards to the floor with a crash.

'Whoops,' Pete said, mirthlessly, stepping aside for one of us to enter the house. Bernard and I stared at each other dumbly, neither sure as to who was going to go in first.

'Pansies,' Pete mumbled, and made his way in first. Bernard followed him.

'Mike Delta from five-nine-two,' I transmitted quickly. 'We've just breached the door to the premises of our last assigned. Going in now.'

'Received,' came the reply.

At least, if they never heard from us again, they'd know where to start looking for our corpses. I followed the others into the apartment.

The door on the far side of the hallway opened and a young, slim black man dressed only in poorly fitting briefs came out of his room, shouting something in a language none of us understood, presumably at the other occupants of the flat.

'Police!' Pete shouted, as if being a six-foot-six Metropolitan Police uniform-clad man didn't make that clear enough. 'We are looking for Stéphane. Please stay where you are.'

The three of us proceeded along the narrow hallway quickly, checking room by room to make sure nobody could run out or vanish out of a window. In the kitchen, we found the man I had seen through the letterbox. He had dropped his towel, and was only moderately successful in preserving his modesty with a small frying pan. Bernard burst out laughing and threw the man his towel.

'Sorry, I didn't mean to laugh,' he said. 'Don't worry, cover yourself up, we just want a chat with you.'

The man accepted the towel, wrapped it around himself and stood there, still holding the frying pan.

'Come with me,' Bernard said, pointing to the door of the kitchen. The man looked confused, and shrugged.

'Please, this way,' I said.

Bernard gently took the frying pan out of the man's hand and led him by the arm out of the kitchen and into the small living room across the hallway.

Bernard's action was the result of many a hard-learned lesson: kitchens are not good places to talk to people who may be about to get arrested. Apart from the frying pan the man had already been holding, I had counted at least six large knives, a meat cleaver and a couple of other potential weapons in the room. I don't know about you, but if I had to choose between being hit with a cast-iron skillet or a sofa cushion, I know what *my* preference is going to be.

'What's your name?' Bernard asked after we had walked into the living room and encouraged the man to sit down in the sofa.

'What?'

'Your name,' Bernard tried again. 'What is it?'

'What?'

'Name,' Bernard continued tirelessly.

'My . . . Name . . . Is . . . Bernard,' he added, pointing at his own chest and prodding his Metvest with every syllable. Then, he pointed at the man. 'Your Name Is . . .?'

'Uh?'

Bernard fished his handcuffs out of their holster.

'If I am not happy that I know who you are, I'm going to arrest you' – he jangled his handcuffs in the air – 'on suspicion of assault, to ascertain your identity properly.'

Suddenly the man remembered his name.

'Charles,' he said. 'My name is Charles.'

'See,' Bernard replied, sardonically. 'That wasn't so hard, was it? Do you have any ID, Charles?'

It appeared that Charles' command of the English language had improved drastically since the beginning of their exchange.

'Yeah, I do,' he said. 'It is in my room.'

'Which one is your room?'

He pointed over his shoulder with his thumb.

Bernard nodded. 'Where in your room?'

'Night stand,' he said. 'Drawer.'

'Would you mind waiting here for me? Is it okay if I go find your ID for you?' Bernard said.

Charles nodded, and I waited around with him until Bernard returned waving a passport. Meanwhile, Pete was standing, wide-legged, blocking the exit of anyone who might try to leave the house and at the same time keeping an eye on the man in briefs.

'When were you born, Charles?' Bernard said.

'September fourteenth, nineteen seventy-three,' he replied.

'Where?'

'Senegal.'

'Where in Senegal?'

'Kaolack.'

'Has anybody ever told you that you don't look a lot like your passport photo?' Bernard asked him, as he passed me the small booklet.

It was one of the old-style passports, where the passport photos were essentially just stapled into place with fancy-looking staples. I looked at the passport closely: it was well worn, but I couldn't really tell whether it was genuine or not; and even if I had been an expert on Senegalese identification documents, I still wouldn't have been able to tell whether the photo had been replaced or not.

Pete had moved further into the flat, and by the sound of things, he was asking similar questions of the other man. A few moments later, Pete brought the second man into the living room. Based on the man's irate tirade, I reasoned that there was nothing wrong with his language skills.

'Flat's clear,' Pete concluded, as he pushed the man brusquely into the living room. 'This guy is a live one.'

'What the hell is this, man?' the man said. 'You broke our fucking door!'

'Why didn't you open up?' Pete asked.

'I was afraid,' he said.

'Of the police?'

'Yeah.'

'Why?'

The man didn't reply.

'Anyway, Charles, I just wanted to . . .' Pete said.

'Wait a minute,' Bernard interrupted, pointing at the man we had found in the kitchen. 'I thought *you* were called Charles'.

'We are both called Charles,' the second man snapped, as if it was the most obvious thing in the world.

We spent the next 20 minutes running both Charleses' details through the police databases. Bernard's Charles came back with a match.

'Have you ever been arrested, Charles?' Bernard said.

Both men immediately shook their heads.

We spent another 45 minutes going back and forth, before reaching the unlikely but apparently accurate conclusion that both these men really were called Charles. And, yes, Bernard's Charles' name really was Charles Ba, but there was another Charles Ba, with the exact same birthday and place of birth, who had been arrested after he had been suspected of a hit-and-run offence in Essex three years prior. It turns out that the Essex-based Charles Ba had a distinctive scar on his face, but our London-based Charles Ba didn't.

You can't make this stuff up.

By the time we had finally cleared up that the two people we were talking to were who they said, the three of us had been in the flat for what felt like roughly an eternity.

'So . . .' Bernard said to our duet of Charleses '. . . we are here to find Stéphane Nguimgo. Do you guys know who he is?'

They shook their heads in perfect unison.

'This house has three bedrooms; there are only two of you here. Who lives in the third bedroom?'

'Nobody,' Pete's Charles volunteered.

'Mate, don't have a laugh. It's quite obvious that someone lives there, there's stuff there.'

'Nobody lives there.'

'Seriously?'

'Nobody. It's a guest room.'

'Do you have a visitor at the moment?'

'No.'

'So there is nobody living in that room?'

'No.'

'Charles, how much rent do you pay?'

'Eh?'

'Rent. The money you pay to live here,' Bernard continued. By now, it was quite clear that both our Charles-named friends spoke absolutely fluent English, but they continued to 'forget' even simple words when it suited them. This happens all the time when questioning people, and can be extremely frustrating. I guess this is why Bernard had taken the lead in talking to the men: I've never met a more patient officer in my life.

'How much do you pay in rent?' he repeated.

'Eighty pounds per week.'

'How long have you been living here?'

'About five years.'

'Do you pay the same?' Bernard turned to the other Charles. He nodded.

'So between the two of you, you pay about a hundred and sixty pounds per week? For this place?'

Charles Ba nodded, but with less conviction this time.

'Mate, this is a pretty good apartment. It's not council, is it?' He shook his head.

'Who is your landlord?'

He shrugged: 'I don't know.'

'You don't know who your landlord is?'

'No.'

'How do you pay him?'

'Cash, every week.'

'How?'

'How?' the man echoed.

'Yes,' Bernard said, and I sensed his patience was beginning to fray. 'Do you meet him somewhere? Does he come here?'

'We send it in the mail.'

'You send cash in the mail?'

'Yes.'

'And it never goes missing in the mail?'

'No.'

'Ever?'

'No.'

'You're lucky, then. I wouldn't generally recommend sending cash in the mail, you know. Not a good idea.'

'To what address do you send the rent money?' Bernard continued.

'I can't remember.'

'Who normally pays the rent?'

'Me.'

'So you've lived here for five years, paid your rent every week, and sent it in the mail every week? So you've written down this address more than two hundred and fifty times, but you can't remember what it is, or who your landlord is?'

'Yes?' the man answered with the most obvious lie of the day yet.

Clearly, there was something really weird going on – the flat we were in was in a pretty dodgy estate, for sure, but the flat itself was pretty nice; it was close to a tube station and local shops. There was no way they were paying £160 per week for this place. Now, if there was a third person involved who shared the rent duties, bringing the total to £240 per week, or about a grand per month in total . . . well, that would still have been cheap, but it sounded more likely.

'I don't believe you,' Bernard said, completely straight-faced. I stifled a chuckle.

'Hey, guys . . .' Pete said, as he walked back into the living room. To my embarrassment, that was the first time I had noticed he had left it in the first place.

There was a small, neatly stacked pile of mail in his hands. I looked at the top envelope in the stack. It was addressed to S. Nguimgo.

'What's this?' I asked Team Charles.

'I don't know,' Pete's Charles lied.

Pete looked through the stack.

'They are bills and letters . . .' he said, as he was going through the stack. 'All addressed to S or Stéphane . . . The newest one was post-marked two days ago, the oldest one about four weeks ago.'

I took a quick look at my wristwatch to confirm the date. Four weeks ago would have been around the beginning of February.

'So here's what I think, guys,' I said. 'There is a third person living here, but it's not Stéphane.'

I looked from Charles to Charles. 'Instead, Stéphane is your landlord, and he comes here at the beginning of every month to pick up his rent and his mail. Is that right?'

Both men remained silent.

I sighed, tearing off a piece of paper from my notebook.

'If you don't want police showing up here every few days, I strongly suggest that you "remember" where Stéphane lives. He's not necessarily in that much trouble, but we *do* need to talk to him urgently. If you know anything, or if you run into him, please call us on this number,' I said, and wrote down '101' in comically large numbers on the pad. 'Or ask *him* to come talk to us at any police station.'

'And now,' Pete says. 'I'm just going to have a quick look in that room where nobody lives, to make sure that nobody is living there at this very moment. Would that be okay?' He looked from Charles to Charles, daring each of them to protest. They didn't.

As we waited, I found myself wondering if Pete really had valid grounds for search. Obviously, we have the right to search for people when we're executing an arrest enquiry, but searching a room where there obviously is nobody home? I figured I'd keep my mouth shut. Still, if Pete felt he could write up an explanation for the search, then it was on him. In his defence, we did have to confirm whether or not our missing person actually lived in this flat, and it would be good for the report to be able to add that extra scrap of information.

Pete returned only a few minutes later and handed me a piece of paper; it was a letter from a mobile phone company.

'Who is Boubacar?' I asked.

One of the Charleses mumbled something.

'Excuse me?' I snapped. I'd lost my patience with these two by now.

We were two hours into a negative arrest enquiry, a process that normally only takes five minutes: you check the house – if the person you're looking for is there, you arrest them and take them to the station; if not, you leave. This was getting a little bit ridiculous.

'It's my brother,' said the Charles who hadn't spoken any English at first.

'Do you know his date of birth?' I asked.

He gave it to me, and I ran Boubacar's details through the computer as well. He came back as wanted in suspicion of several counts of fraud, all committed in Birmingham.

'What does your brother do for a living, Charles?' I asked.

He shrugged, and I tried to encourage him to tell me where his brother might be, but Charles claimed to know absolutely nothing. Eventually, I gave up.

I looked up at Pete, then across to Bernard.

'Are we done here?' I asked. The uniform-clad pair turned away, in perfect synchrony. I knew they felt the same as me: we had wasted a monumental amount of time and effort on a completely fruitless arrest enquiry, on a day when the borough was seriously short on staff.

Ridiculous.

As I started to leave, Pete's Charles piped up.

'Hey, who is going to pay for the door?' he said.

'You have home insurance, don't you?' I answered, and started digging around in my Metvest. Pete tapped me on the shoulder and shoved the flyer I was looking for into my hand with a grin. I was not particularly surprised to discover that Pete, who had a passion for kicking doors open, carried on him the information leaflet we hand out in these situations.

'Next time,' I said to the Charleses, handing over the flyer, 'when the police knock on your door, try opening. It's cheaper.'

Feeling despondent, we started walking down the four flights. That was a total of three officers times three hours – so, 12 hours of police constable time – wasted, for nothing.

However, before we fully made it to the bottom of the stairs, our bad moods were lifted: a group of youths had been seen 'fighting with sticks' (that means baseball or cricket bats, usually) in a nearby park. There was no way we weren't going to be the first officers on scene.

'Show six-eight,' Bernard shouted into his radio as he ran towards the Panda.

'Show eight-seven,' I echoed, not a second later, as we leapt into the caged van, before flicking the lights and sirens on, following the Astra to the location at high speed.

A shot to the heart

I had reached the halfway point in my shift, and it had been completely and utterly dead all morning. I'm sure quite a few of my colleagues would disagree with me when I say this, but I much prefer *busy*.

Officially, our shifts are about nine hours long, with a one-hour overlap with the next shift. This means, sometimes you might be dismissed earlier, because the next shift has managed to get their act together quickly; other times, you're working for ten hours straight – or much worse, because you end up with an arrest minutes before the shift is meant to end.

Don't get me wrong; the overtime is a delicious sprinkling of cold, hard, additional queenheads sitting in my bank account, but it is also properly knackering.

However, the reason I love busy shifts, is that one finds oneself looking at one's watch, only to realise that the shift ends in 20 minutes. When a whole day flies by as if it's nothing, it's hard not to enjoy work. Naturally, 'tis not always so . . .

Monday mornings can be pretty bleak during the cold snaps that come in the midst of winter. This is typically when the office-bound social services folk realise that the people they are looking after haven't been in touch for a while. Instead of checking up on their wards themselves, they'll call the police. Then, one of us will be despatched to a house or flat somewhere. Frequently, there's absolutely nothing wrong other than someone has forgotten to pay their phone bill. At less fortunate times, we might find an elderly, infirm or mentally unstable resident a bit worse for wear, possibly in the progress of conducting a mutually beneficial business merger (or a fluid-fibre exchange, if you will) with the carpet on the living-room floor or the mattress in their bedroom.

What made this Monday particularly unpleasant was that I was feeling a little bit hung over. My quiet Sunday-night trip to the pub had turned into a tequila-slamming headache-fest of gorilla-sized proportions. I would have felt this to be irresponsible on a school night, if it hadn't been for the fact that Sunday's early shift had been so awful that tequilas were completely necessary and strictly medicinal.

As soon as I rolled out of the gate to the police station on the Sunday morning, I was despatched at great haste to the scene of a freshly expired 18-year-old student, who had been found by his now-in-need-of-some-serious-therapy university housemates. Apparently (and I'm not a coroner, so the 'apparently' means that I can't really say for sure, but my untrained eyes made the following conclusions) he'd decided to put a full stop to his not-even-really-started life in a particularly gruesome way that left his student halls room covered in claret. My shift was punctuated (I like to think of my lunch-breaks as a semi-colon: longer than a comma, but with a light dusting of suspense at what might be coming next) with a sizeable kebab that smelled worse than the aforementioned 18-year-old. As disgusting as my mid-shift refuelling choice might have been, I was still dismayed that the eating of it was rudely interrupted by my radio despatching me to yet another sudden death: another absolute tragedy where it appears that a woman around my age died of drowning following a freak falling-over-in-the-bathtub incident. Somehow she had not been found until ten days later.

Anyway, today was another day. I had spent the morning on a marked motorbike. It's unusual for us to do response duties on a motorbike – mostly response duties are carried out in a car. Patrol taskings, on the other hand, can be fulfilled by pedal bike or car. Motorbikes tend to be reserved for traffic and robbery duties. However, a significant number of the response cars were out of action (otherwise known as 54'd[66]). The shift skipper figured they might as well try to put as many uniforms on the streets as they could, so, since Robbery were using their Q-car instead of the bikes, he sent me out with the keys to a shiny new BMW motorbike.

I really like being on a police bike (or a 'Solo', as we call them). If you think a police car on lights-and-sirens is a quick way to get around in London, you've never tried riding a 1200cc touring bike with blue-and-yellow battenburg markings, a frankly unnecessarily loud siren, and lots of flashing blue lights through rush-hour traffic. I won't lie: it's good fun.

I'd been assigned to a part of the borough where there had been a spate of thefts from vehicles – sat-nav units, for the most part – so I was casually cruising along the edge of the tasking area. However, a light drizzle earlier in the day, along with a distinct nip in the air, meant that the roads were empty: nobody in their right mind wanted to leave their nice cosy house.

'Mike Delta three-seven,' my radio broadcast. At first, I didn't respond: three-seven is not an oft-used call sign, and I didn't think

---

[66] Form 54 is filled in when a Met vehicle has to be taken off the road for any reason: anything from a broken indicator bulb to a blown engine results in a car being 54'd, and it can't be taken out until the problem is fixed by a Met-approved mechanic.

I'd ever been issued that designation before (nor do I think I've been issued it since).

'Go ahead,' I replied eventually, when I realised they were talking to me.

'The next borough over has had a serious incident; an IC3 male, aged around fifteen, has been stabbed in the chest, apparently. They're stretched for staff, and need someone to help land the HEMS[67] helicopter. Are you free to head over?'

'Sure thing,' I replied, flicking my blues on. 'Give me five minutes and the exact location, please?'

'I'll send it to your MDT,' the operator said.

'Er, I haven't got one,' I said. 'I'm on a bike.'

'Of course you are. My apologies,' the operator transmitted, before instructing me to switch to the spare channel in order to fill me in on the incident over the radio instead.

As the operator gave me the details, I clocked that the incident had happened in the opposite end of the borough. In effect, that meant a blue-light run from my location, all the way across town. Once I'd been briefed, and had my marching orders, I switched the bike radio to the despatch channel of the borough I was going to. As soon as I switched, I realised they were dealing with pandemonium over there. There were dozens of incidents in progress and the radio channel was absolute chaos.

'Foxtrot Bravo receiving Mike Delta three-seven?' I transmitted as soon as there was a tiny gap in radio traffic

'Go ahead.'

'Just to confirm I'm running from Mike Delta to the location to assist HEMS landing.'

'Received, thanks. Let us know when you get there.'

Travelling along the dual carriageway connecting the two

---

[67] Helicopter Emergency Medical Service: the London Air Ambulance charity

boroughs at speeds of anything between zero and 90 miles per hour – whatever the fastest safe speed was given the circumstances, bearing in mind that the whole stretch of road has 40 or 50 limits – I wondered whether I'd be able to even beat HEMS to the location. It sounded pretty unlikely.

Sure, on a high-powered motorcycle it sort of *feels* like you're flying through traffic, but HEMS is *actually* flying, and usually at about 150mph. I'm pretty sure the BMW K1200 could reach 150mph if I really pushed it, but my route had pesky obstacles like cars, roundabouts, buildings and pedestrians, whereas the ghetto-bird simply skips over everything. It was going to be an interesting little race, for sure.

'Foxtrot Bravo, Foxtrot Bravo, Helimed two-seven Alpha requesting talk-through with Mike Delta three-seven,' my radio sung with the HEMS co-pilot's almost satirically polite voice.

The police helicopter is known as India 99 (if there is more than one helicopter in the air at a given time, their call signs are India 98, India 97, etc). This wasn't the first time I'd noticed that a heli-pilot has an outrageously posh accent. Perhaps it's a prerequisite to be allowed to fly rotary-winged aircraft above the fair city of London? The other thing the heli-pilots do rather splendidly is absolutely immaculate radio protocol. I quite like it when they butt into our radio channels; in their extreme clarity, they put the rest of us to shame. On the flipside, if any of our police officers followed perfect protocol when on response duties, they'd be the butt of every joke.

The heli-pilot's timing for talk-through was perfect: I had just pulled the bike onto the centre stand having arrived at the location where the helicopter was going to land. All in all, the blue-light run had taken just over seven minutes – not bad for covering around six and a half miles. If my maths skills don't elude me, that meant I had an average speed of just over 50mph – not too shabby at all, I thought, as I mentally patted myself on the back. It's hard not to feel a little bit like a superhero when you manage to beat a helicopter through rush-hour traffic.

Across from the park was a large, low-slung warehouse. Parked up outside were three cars: one was a paramedic's, the other two were police cars. I could hear sounds coming from the warehouse, so presumed that that was where the victim was.

'Go ahead, Helimed two-seven Alpha. Talk-through authorised, the channel is yours,' the operator said, giving the helicopter permission to talk to me directly over the Foxtrot Delta despatch channel.

'Thank you, Foxtrot Bravo. Mike Delta three-seven, our ETA is four minutes, we are running from a training mission outside the M25. Is the landing location ready?' the HEMS helicopter asked.

'Negative, Helimed two-seven,' I transmitted, a little bit disappointed. I thought I had somehow beaten the helicopter flying in from the Royal London – in reality they had been much further away. 'You are landing in a small park next to the incident; I am at location now, but there are some people on location. I'll clear them and confirm.'

'Thank you, Mike Delta three-seven,' the chopper crew said. 'Foxtrot Bravo, thanks for the talk-through. Helimed two-seven Alpha out.'

I unplugged myself from the bike radio (something you remember to do automatically after nearly ripping your ear off a few times), left my helmet on the bike's rear-view mirror, and moved my personal radio from my jacket pocket to the clip on the front of my Metvest. I hadn't yet changed the channel on my personal radio to the official channel, so I fiddled with it as I approached the two people in the park.

'Hi there,' I said to two men who were seated on a bench at the edge of the small green. One of them shuffled away immediately, grunting something as he left. He glanced back at me defiantly, as if daring me to challenge him. Normally, that's a good indication that they're carrying something they shouldn't be, but I wasn't on a drugs mission: I was there to clear the park, and he was doing my job for me. Thank you, sir!

'Hello,' the other man said. He had an open can by his feet – cider, I think – and was trying to hide it with his leg.

'We have had a bit of an incident,' I started, realising that I didn't really know exactly what had happened, beyond the fact that someone had been stabbed. All I knew was that if he was in need of the air ambulance, it must be pretty serious.

'So?' the man said.

'We're going to be landing a helicopter in this space, and it'll be too dangerous for you to be here,' I said. 'I'm going to have to ask you to leave the area.'

'Aha?' he said.

'Please move, sir,' I said, pointing towards the gate of the low fence surrounding the park.

'No,' he said, simply.

I blinked.

'Sorry?'

'No. I have a right to be here. Not moving,' he said, and wrapped his threadbare coat tighter around him.

'Uhm . . . *Yes*. You're going to have to move,' I replied. 'I'm going to need this space. A helicopter is going to land here,' I repeated, in an exercise of mind-numbing futility.

The man looked back at me, cocking his head slightly. I stole a furtive glance at my watch.

'I'm really sorry, but I don't have time for this. You're *really* going to have to go now,' I said.

'No,' he said, glancing over my shoulder. I looked behind me. The man who had left us was standing near my motorcycle, looking at it closely.

I sighed.

'You have ten seconds to get out of this park,' I said. 'Someone is seriously hurt, and we are going to need an ambulance helicopter to land here so they can save his life.'

'I pay my taxes,' the man said. 'What right do you have to force me to move?'

'I'm not forcing you,' I said, doing my best to avoid a confrontation. 'I'm asking you very, very nicely if you could pretty please move somewhere else. I don't even care if you take your drink with you – I won't take it off you. I really need this space and it's going to be dangerous to be here very soon.'

'I'm not moving,' the man said. 'I fought for my country, you know. You can't tell me to do anything. I know my rights.'

There are times when I rather enjoy discussions about the law with people who don't believe they have to do what I say. This was not one of those times. I glanced nervously at my watch for a second time and realised that if their estimation was any good (and it usually is), the helicopter was going to arrive any second.

'If you were hurt, would you want the helicopter to come and rescue you?'

'Yes.'

'So what would happen if someone refused to let the helicopter land?'

'I don't know,' he said, twitching a little. 'I don't care.'

I began to wonder whether the guy might be suffering from psychological issues of some sort.

'Don't you think you are being a little bit unreasonable?'

'No. Fuck off. I like this park,' he said, reaching for his cider. The only time our eyes met throughout the whole conversation was then, as he took a huge gulp of cider. He held the can up, as if to say 'cheers', and drank again. I regretted telling him that I wasn't going to take his can of cider off him, because my usual course of action would be to pour it out and send him on his way.

'Move!' I said. 'Now. I will explain everything to you afterwards, if you like, but this helicopter is going to arrive any second.'

'No,' he said, simply, before sucking down the rest of the cider, picking up a new can from the Tesco bag behind the bench and starting to tap the top of the can with his fingertips. He opened it slowly, with deliberate movements, and took another sip, all without acknowledging me with as much as a glance.

'Please?' I tried.

'Why don't you piss off?' he said.

By now I could hear the helicopter in the distance, and as I glanced behind me, I saw that another police car had pulled up next to the three cars that were already outside the warehouse.

'Seriously, if you don't fuck off out of this park right now, I'm going to have to remove you by force,' I exploded, with a spectacular lack of professionalism.

'I'll have you for assault,' the man said, with a small shrug.

Two officers stepped out of the police car. One of them waved at me, whilst the other – a sergeant – went straight into the warehouse. I waved back to the constable and indicated for him to come to me.

As the constable – a slender-looking chap in an immaculately ironed uniform – approached, I shouted the details of the situation to him: 'Helicopter is nearly here. This guy is refusing to move. Give me a hand.'

I turned back to the man in the park.

'Okay, I've warned you several times. You can hear the helicopter. I don't really care if it lands on top of you, but it delays the paramedics, so you're now going to leave the park.'

'Fuck off,' he said, simply.

'You heard my colleague, William, we need to land this helicopter now, or our injured friend could die,' the officer said.

I read his nametag: Police Constable Frost.

'You heard *me*,' William replied. Then slowly and deliberately, turning between the two of us, he added: 'Fuck. Off.'

I heard the unmistakeable clicking sound of a baton being racked next to me.

'Gis a hand,' Constable Frost said, before grabbing William by the arm. I leapt into action, and tried to secure his other arm.

William tried to hang on to the bench with his hands, but Frost slammed his baton into the metal a couple of inches away from his fingers with a loud metallic crash that sent vibrations all the way through the bench. He hissed, 'The next one goes on your fingers – come on, stop fucking about.'

Wisely, William decided to let go of the bench, and the two of us policemen dragged him along the grass towards the gate, with him shouting 'Police brutality!' 'Murder!' and 'Someone take a picture! See what they are doing to me!' all the way.

A few people stopped along the edges of the park to look on, attracted as much by the helicopter that was lowering out of the sky as the man shouting bloody murder.

I looked over to my bike. William's friend had left, but I saw that my motorcycle helmet had left with him. *Great.*

At the edge of the park, we let William go.

'If you try to enter the park again, I will handcuff you to this railing,' Frost said, pointing with his baton to the metal fence next to the gate.

'I want to complain! Police brutality!' William shouted, beside himself with anger and frustration. 'You owe me a cider, you bastards!'

'You want to complain? No problem,' Frost said. 'Here, use my phone.'

The constable handed over a waterproof-looking orange-and-blue mobile that was so desperately unfashionable that it had to be a work phone.

'The number you want is one-zero-one,' he said.

I left Frost with the man, and took a few steps into the small park just as the helicopter landed in the seemingly-impossibly-small space. Before it had even fully come to rest on the ground, a paramedic and a doctor hopped out. I pointed to the warehouse, and they nodded to me before running in a helicopter-blade-avoiding half-crouch towards the warehouse, small suitcases of medical equipment in hand.

The co-pilot gave me a quick thumbs-up as the chopper touched down.

I looked over at Frost. He was standing with William, who was speaking into the phone, lamenting his violent eviction from the park. When he finally rang off, he gave the phone back to Frost and stumbled away.

'Old William's normally harmless,' Frost said to me, as I walked up to him. 'But he is rather paranoid.'

'Did he file a complaint?' I asked.

'Yeah, I think they directed him to the police station to file a formal complaint and to do the paperwork. That's where he's headed now, I believe,' Frost said with a shrug.

He stuck a hand out.

'I'm Jeremy,' he said.

'Matt,' I replied. 'Nice to meet you. Thanks for your help.'

'No worries. We have to deal with William quite often. He's a regular on the borough. Keeps saying he knows his rights but then doesn't act as if he knows any of his responsibilities,' he shrugged. 'He's good as gold most of the time, but he does a bit of shoplifting and can't get it into his head that we can search him. He even accused one of the WPCs, Sandra, of rape the last time he was arrested, which caused a bit of palaver.'

'Shit, how did that end?' I asked, as we were walking towards the warehouse together.

'Sandra helped when he refused to let himself be fingerprinted. It got quite messy, but it was all on CCTV in custody, so it won't go anywhere. He just seems to like complaining about us whenever he can.'

'Bloody hell,' I said.

'Yeah, it's a pain in the arse. And of course, they have to investigate any allegations, but it's such a waste of time. Better make sure you write this up carefully, Matt,' he said, before he excused himself.

'Thanks, buddy,' I called after him, and I walked into the warehouse.

Whenever we use force – whether it's actual force or just a threat – we have to write it up and justify it carefully, whether the write up is for an EAB[68], another form or just a pocketbook entry. I always keep careful notes anyway, but Jeremy's warning was welcome nonetheless. It often feels as if what we write down only gets scrutinised when someone complains about use of force. But, I suppose, this is rightly so.

Inside the warehouse, I was met by quite the drama.

The kid was still on the warehouse floor. The HEMS doctor had just finished opening his chest with a rib spreader – a device that wouldn't be out of place in a medieval torture museum. A device that also gruesomely accurately named: a rib spreader spreads ribs. I stood watching in the background as the doctor shoved both his hands into the gaping hole in the boy's chest.

The paramedics who had arrived in their car were standing by, ready to jump in if they were needed.

'What the hell happened here?' I asked one of them. 'How old is he?'

'He looks about fifteen, but we haven't been able to ID him

[68] Evidence and Action Book

yet,' one of the paramedics replied. 'He was stabbed in the chest, and it looks like they nicked his heart. The trauma guys are trying to stop the bleed before whisking him off to the Royal.'

'Did they catch the suspect?' I asked the paramedic. The sergeant, who'd arrived with Jeremy and was standing on the other side of me, jumped in with a reply.

'Not yet. But we know who he is; one of our guys recognised him on the CCTV footage. The sus is only about sixteen, but he's a known gang member. Nothing but trouble. The Borough Support Unit are going around to find him,' the skipper explained, without ever taking his eyes off the victim. 'This poor bastard had better pull through; I'm really not in the mood for a murder today.'

When he finally tore his eyes away from the live-action medical drama in front of us, he turned to me. 'We were a bit thin on the ground today; your help is most appreciated. I imagine I'll be the one dealing with William's complaint at our end later, so make sure you've got your altercation written up carefully.'

'Yeah,' I replied. 'Jeremy said as much. Complains a lot, does he?'

The skipper only laughed.

'Hey, Delito,' a voice sounded behind me.

I turned around to see Jeremy had returned.

'Think quick! Present for you,' he said, and tossed something towards me. I caught the item before I'd even realised it was my motorcycle helmet.

'Where'd you find it?' I asked him, feeling very grateful. I had been worrying about all the hoops I would have to go through to get a helmet brought to me from the police station in order for me to be able to ride my Solo back to base.

'The pub.'

'What?'

'The guy who took it. He nicks stuff all the time, and always sells it at the pub down the road.'

'How did you know who took it? He left before you arrived?'

'William told me,' he said. 'I made him a deal. I told him the payment for borrowing my phone was telling me who his friend was.'

'And that worked?'

'You've got your helmet, don't you?' Jeremy said.

'Ha! Thanks,' I said, shaking his hand.

'We had one of the probationers nick him for theft. They're going to need a statement from you about the helmet when you have a chance.'

'No problem; looks like I'll be doing a lot of writing today anyway – what's an extra couple of MG-11s?'

I jotted a quick note on my hand to remind myself to write a witness statement about the incident.

Behind us was a flurry of activity as the paramedics and helicopter crew prepared the victim for a helicopter ride. I left them to it and walked back to my motorbike, helmet in hand.

The memory of the paramedic, elbow-deep in the kid's blood right there on the dirty warehouse floor sent a chill down my spine.

I started the heavy BMW motorbike and began to make my way back to the police station to spend some quality time with a cup of coffee, a black ballpoint pen and a ream of paper.

As I was waiting at a stoplight, I found myself crossing my fingers, hoping that the kid would survive the next few hours.

He didn't.

Ambushed in the Riots

The briefing for the late shift was nothing out of the ordinary. At least, in the same way that strolling to work and finding Elvis in a tap-dancing competition with Chairman Mao, accompanied by the cast of *Glee* playing a Latin American-flavoured cover of Culture Club's 'Do You Really Want to Hurt Me' would be nothing out of the ordinary.

The briefing is usually at 2 p.m., which means that most of my colleagues show up at work around 1 p.m. to shower, change into their uniforms, read the day's briefing and emails, and then stroll over to the briefing room for a few rounds of pre-shift banter.

Usually.

Today, everybody had arrived at the briefing room more than an hour before it was due to start. The room was chock-a-block with chatter.

A few days earlier, in Tottenham, police officers had shot a suspected gang leader in a minicab.

'Damn right he deserved to be shot, he had a fucking gun,' one of my colleagues said. 'They need to start understanding that if you're carrying a gun, you're likely to get shot, whether it's by another gang, or by us.'

'Pipe down, Charlie,' Jay responded. He was speaking from

265

experience; he'd been a firearms officer for many years. 'It's never that simple, mate. I heard on the news that they found an unloaded gun in a sock. You can't just go around shooting people if they don't have a gun that's even ready to use. It's insane that we're even talking about this – one of our colleagues was shot. It's the gung-ho attitude that will get us in trouble, my friend.'

We were all shocked about the shooting of a police officer, but thankfully he'd survived.

'Ah, fuck off, you has-been,' Charlie fired back at Jay. He followed up with a smile, but he was a fraction too late.

Being called a 'has-been' clearly didn't sit well with Jay – anger flared across his face.

Jay and Charlie were old friends. Like all of us, they love a spot of banter. Everybody knew that Jay had decided to stand down from being an authorised firearms officer. However, not many people knew why. All that *was* universally known was that Jay doesn't like talking about it.

Banter. It's part of the job. You can't deal with the things we do day in, day out without having an outlet; black humour, practical jokes, making a bit of fun of each other, and the occasional bit of rough-housing comes with the job. It's part of the fabric that weaves us together as a team. We spend a lot of time wrestling on the floor with smelly criminals, running after scoundrels and dealing with death. A playful punch on the shoulder, a hug or some gentle ribbing here and there is the lubrication that keeps the machine running. Just make sure you don't tell the SMT[69]; they'd send us all on How to Be Nice to Each Other courses.

The importance of a strong team spirit is one reason why we felt all the more uneasy in the briefing room that morning. When the joking grinds to a halt, we get caught in a vicious cycle: more

[69] Senior Management Team

tension causes less banter, causes more tension – this shift was off to a truly rotten start.

I was glad when the briefing finally started.

'Read the briefing in your own time, at your own pace,' the skipper barked, 'but the summary is this: it's messy out there, and it's going to be rough for a few days.'

The Metropolitan Police intel branch was red-hot with tips received via telephone, found on Internet forums, and pilfered from social-networking sites – they all pointed to all-out riots.

The skipper leaned forward over his little speaker's podium, casting a long look across the room. He looked evil in the red glow from the projector in the darkened briefing room.

'Ladies and gents, stay very alert: the gang who lost their boss to a police bullet say they want the lives of two Metropolitan Police officers in retaliation for the shooting . . .' He paused. 'We're particularly worried about the specificity: normally, threats are non-specific. This time, intel suggests that they are planning a definite hit. I won't lie to you; it's going to be bloody dangerous for a while. However, we've got lots of extra resources on the ground, including extra Trojan[70] units.'

He stopped and took a sip from his water bottle. I looked at my colleagues; they were glued to his every word. It was going to be tough to be a police officer in our borough for the foreseeable future.

'As you know, we're short-staffed,' the skipper said, and then grinned. 'I hate recruitment, so try to stay in one piece, all right?'

A wave of laughter spread throughout the room and some of the tension dissolved.

Charlie slapped Jay on the shoulder, and got a shrug and a smile in return – an apology accepted.

---

[70] Specialist Firearms Officers (SFOs)

It's episodes like this that remind me why some of the skippers are promoted ahead of others – sometimes, all it takes to save the day is for someone to just reel the team back in, to put us back on the right track. We were ready, now, to deal with the outside world.

'No single-crewing tonight, folks. Be extra vigilant, and don't hesitate to call in help if you aren't sure about something. I'd rather have to send two or three cars to a call and have everyone go home at the end of the shift, than be stuck in A&E with one of you for the rest of the night,' the skipper added, scanning the room.

'Right, get out of my face. Happy hunting,' he finished.

And with that, we were sent out onto the meaner-than-usual streets of London.

In several parts of the borough, there had been stirrings of civil unrest: people had been seen gathering in alleys. Many shops on the high streets had boarded up their windows with plywood.

We were instructed to stay well clear of any problem spots. They were to be left to the Level Ones. The Level Ones were operating on separate channels from us, and it was made clear to us that we'd face disciplinary action if we listened in. 'Any relevant information will be circulated on working channels,' a sternly worded email from the top brass reminded us.

Public order training comes in three levels – three, two and one:

Level Three is the basic level of public order skills used for policing large events, such as football games, official state visits, and anywhere where the police have to work as large teams and face large groups of members of the public – it covers all officers.

Level Two officers are trained to a much higher degree, including shield tactics, dealing with extremely violent people, rapid-entry techniques (including stuff like breaking down doors), search tactics and much, much more. When you think 'riot police', the people that spring to mind are probably the Level Two guys.

Level One officers have roughly the same training curriculum as for Level Two, but they have to repeat their training every six weeks or so, and are generally deployed to a 'support unit' full-time.

Our job that night would be to look after all the 'normal' police tasks (if anything could be called normal on a day like this).

I was posted with Jay – our ex-firearms officer – as Mike Delta 40. It's an unusual call sign; we don't tend to use 40, but this was an unusual day. There were a huge number of extra resources on duty; a lot of the officers who generally while away their days shuffling bits of paper around had dusted off their uniforms. In some cases, our extra show of force would prove more entertaining than preventative: officers who had gained 30lb since the last time they had worn their stab vests looked anything but digni-fied as they tried to wrestle their way into a corset-like Kevlar.

The extra manpower also meant that we used a lot of cars we don't normally use: a fleet of hire-cars were brought in to help ferry us around from place to place without standing out like a sore blue-lights-and-sirens-equipped thumb.

Today, Mike Delta 40 was a hideous burgundy Ford Mondeo Q-car, usually used by the robbery squad. At least it had lights and sirens, as opposed to most of the hire cars.

'I'll drive,' Jay said with a groan, after he'd spotted the car we had been assigned.

I was fine with that. In theory, Jay and I are both advanced drivers, trained to the same high standard. I'd like to think I'm an above-average wheelman, even in the context of the ridiculously well-trained advanced drivers amongst the Metropolitan Police.

Realistically, however, I'm probably a distinctly average advanced driver.

Jay, on other hand, used to be the driver on firearms callouts; he has no doubt spent a hell of a lot more time on long blue-light runs than me. There was also something about that shift that was giving me the creeps, and I was more than happy to hand over some responsibility – *any* responsibility. Not having to drive seemed like a good start.

First up, we attended to a couple of simple-to-resolve calls.

My feeling of dread began to dissipate a little.

After about five hours of relatively easy jobs (including – believe it or not – saving a kitten stuck in a tree), we decided to head back to the police station for a quick coffee.

We'd nearly made back, when things got a little bit more interesting . . .

My radio lurched into action: 'We've just spotted a group of about twenty youths, some of them carrying backpacks. They all have their faces covered. Most of them are carrying sticks,' it told me. 'We're in an unmarked car, observing from a safe distance,' the radio continued.

Instead of pulling into the police station, Jay pulled up next to the gates. We stayed in the car to listen to the radio transmission in progress, both trying to figure out who was radioing in; I didn't recognise his voice and he sounded nervous. He also failed to identify himself before transmitting, which was curious. Radio protocol becomes such second nature that it becomes unthinkable to radio up without first going through the recipe of identifying yourself and asking for permission to use the airwaves.

'Last caller, you are not coming up in my system. Please identify,' the CAD operator shot back. I looked over at Jay, and he shrugged.

'Oh, eh, sorry,' said the radio, and went quiet again, briefly.

'They're coming our way. We have to get out of here,' it continued.

'Last caller, get yourself to safety, then identify immediately. Mike Delta three out,' a familiar voice cut in. Mike Delta 3 is the chief inspector, a person you would *never* hear on the radio unless something truly grievous was going on. Hell, I didn't even know he was *issued* with a radio.

'Mike Delta receiving one-zero-eight,' a new voice joined in.

'One-zero-eight, go,' the CAD operator replied.

'Last transmitting was five-two-two-eight, Smith. He's the special I've got with me. It's his first shift,' the voice continued.

I raised an eyebrow, and glanced over at Jay who met my gaze with an identical eyebrow-raised-expression. We both burst into laughter.

A special constable deciding to take his first shift as a police officer on a night when there are riots going on? Talk about baptism of fire! Having said that, one-zero-eight is Singh, a solid, veteran officer. I couldn't think of a safer pair of hands if I tried.

'We're on Church Street, moving away as quickly as we can. I think the group spotted our radios lighting up when someone transmitted,' Singh concluded.

The radios: they're a blessing most of the time – they can be the lifeline that keeps us out of a lot of serious trouble. But there's no denying, they're bulky, and have a nasty tendency to ruin any plain-clothes work you're trying to do. The displays and the status light might as well be a bright beacon saying, 'Hey! We're cops! If you're up to no good, this is a good time to start running!'

'Okay, is everybody accounted for?' the CAD operator asked.

'Yes, yes, we're out of harm's way,' Singh replied.

'Good. All units, please avoid Church Street for now, we'll send the Borough Support Unit to take a closer look,' the CAD operator transmitted.

'Mike Delta receiving serial bravo-alpha-five-five-five,' a new voice chimed out.

'Go ahead, BA five-five-five.'

'I know you wanted BSU on this, but we're a Level One serial here, and we're just around the corner. Shall we head over as well?' the voice continued.

'Yes, yes, please deploy and keep us posted,' the CAD operator said, and continued to liaise with the Borough Support Unit to get a couple of more carriers over to the group who seemed keen to start their own little riot.

'It's really going to suck to be them,' Jay laughed drily.

'Mike Delta four-zero receiving,' another CAD operator interrupted.

'Go ahead,' I transmitted.

'Switch to spare, please,' the operator requested.

I reached for my radio and switched to the spare channel, leaving the despatch channel free to organise units for the violent disorder incident.

'Mike Delta receiving four-zero,' I transmitted on the new channel.

'Hi, Matt,' the operator said, leaving the formal tone of the main channel behind. Technically, radio protocol is meant to apply on all channels, but it always sounds really weird when people go through the full patter, especially when you know the person on the other end of the radio and there's only half a dozen people listening in.

'Hey, Samantha. Busy?'

'You bet. Are you guys dealing with anything?'

'Nope, just stopped for a cuppa, but we can be free.'

'Great. You're double-crewed, right?'

'Yeah, I'm with Jay.'

'Remind me of his shoulder number?'

'It's four-eight-three. That's four-eight-three.'

'Great, noted. We've just had an abandoned call from a phone box. It reported shouting, and what sounded like a man beating up a woman over on the Blankenship Estate, near the playground. We couldn't get any more information, and nobody is picking up the phone at the booth. CCTV has no coverage. Can you zip over and have a peek?'

'Yeah, of course. On the hurry-up?'

'Yes, please, on an I-grade. Is your Mobile Data Terminal working?'

'No, sorry, we're in a Q-car. No MDT. I know where it is, though. What's the CAD number?'

'CAD seven-two-eight-nine-two of today.'

'Wicked, we'll take a look'

'Thanks, sweets; say hi to Jay from me. Out.'

I turned to Jay.

'Samantha says hi,' I said.

'Yeah, I heard that. How very nice,' he said, sardonically. Sam and Jay used to date a few years back, but that came to a rather acrimonious end, which – much like Jay's exit from the AFOs – nobody knows much about.

Jay spun the wheel and pulled away from the gates.

'Next left,' I said a few minutes later.

'Then it should be the third or fourth right, right?' Jay grunted in reply.

We pulled up outside Blankenship, in a weird little deserted car park. There were walls in front of us and to our left, and on the third side there was a hedge and the playground Sam had mentioned.

The whole area was completely dead.

Jay leaned forward over the wheel and peered up into the council blocks. Blankenship is not one of the roughest estates we have on the borough, but it's on the edge of an area known for a large amount of gang activity. It has more than its fair share of stabbings, and police aren't exactly welcomed with fanfares, scones and tea.

'I don't like this,' Jay said, sucking his teeth and reaching for his radio.

'Show Mike Delta four-zero on location of our last assigned,' he stated, adhering to a spot of routine that may well have saved our lives.

'I don't like this at all,' he repeated, after we'd had confirmation of our transmission.

'There's the phone,' I said, pointing to the booth. It was just in front of the hedge. All of the windows of the box were smashed, and the rest of it was covered so thoroughly in graffiti that I found myself surprised that the box actually still worked well enough to place a 999 call. There's something to say for the engineering BT puts into its iconic red boxes.

'I can't hear anything. Can you?' Jay said.

I rolled my window down ever so slightly to have a listen.

'Nope, I can't hear any—'

I was interrupted by the smashing of the window next to my head. Pain shot through my neck, and out of the corner of my eye I saw someone grab for the door next to me. They pulled the handle hard; the whole car rocked. It was locked. It always is. I lock my door out of habit, whether I'm on duty or not.

I turned towards my window and saw four people outside. One of the dark shadows had reached his hand inside the window they had just smashed with a brick, and was attempting to reach for the door lock. He was so close that I could smell his arm: a musky tang of earth, cigarettes and cheap laundry detergent. For a second, I thought about how odd it was that I was sitting there, smelling the arm of someone who had just broken the window that shielded me from the elements.

I snapped out of my shock and looked down at my hand. I

had picked up the spare battery for my radio. I didn't waste any more time and brought it down on his hand. Hard. The young man yelped in pain and pulled away from the door, before running towards the back of the car; his friends did the same.

I sensed something happening beside me, and turned to Jay.

Or rather, I turned to the space where Jay should have been.

The men – boys, really – had opened the door on his side of the car, and were trying to drag him out of the driver-side door. He was still wearing his seatbelt, and the nylon straps digging into his lap, neck and shoulder were the only things keeping him in the car.

Our in-car MDTs have huge 'emergency' buttons on them in case we need help. I reached for the space in the centre console where the button was—where the button *would have been*, if this car had had an MDT installed. I lost precious seconds registering there was no help to be had from the dashboard, other than the button to switch on the car's flashing lights. I pressed it, activating the blue lights that are hidden in the grille at the front of the car and as blue LEDs in the reversing lights at the back. Jay, in his struggles, was pressing on the steering wheel, and managed to turn on the car's sirens as well. Every time he bumped into the horn buttons built into the wheel, the tone of the sirens changed from one melody to another.

The small, darkened area was suddenly lit up with stroboscopic blues. The deafening cacophony of the sirens echoed off the walls.

Somewhere in all of this, I found my senses and pressed the red button on my radio.

'Urgent assistance required,' I shouted.

I grabbed the door-release handle and bounced out of the car, reaching for my baton with one hand.

As I stood up, a lap-full of glass rained down off me. Glass was everywhere. I could feel it sticking into my shoulders where it had dug its way under my Metvest. It was gnawing into my sides. My eye felt . . . odd . . . but I had but one thing on my mind: helping Jay, and then getting the hell out of there.

I started moving to the back of the car, continuing my frenetic, shouted monologue into my radio: 'We're under attack!' I shouted. 'Six males, maybe more.'

A few of the group who'd been attacking us had been scared off by the sirens. By the time I had staggered around to Jay's side of the car, there were just three left.

Jay was half-hanging out of the vehicle, and one of the men was making to kick him. In excruciating slow motion, I saw the attacker bring his leg forward hard.

'Get away from him,' I shouted, and raised my baton to strike. There was one man between Jay and myself. He saw my stick and began to move out of the way, but I was not in the mood to find out whether he was planning to run off; anything or anybody between me and Jay was going to get a whack with the length of freshly-racked extendible steel I had clutched between my fingers.

I swung at the man with my baton. I couldn't hear it, but I felt a crunching as the brushed steel impacted with the lower arm he had thrown up to defend himself.

I could see Jay's head bouncing up, and helplessly falling back down again, as yet another boot connected. One of the men was holding him by his arm, still trying to drag him out of the car, as the other kicked him.

'Get back,' I shouted, on autopilot – 'get back' is the universal fighting call that gets drilled into you in officer safety training.

I brought the baton down on the first man again. This time, he lifted his other arm. My baton connected with something metal. It was a pole. He was holding a short length of scaffolding or piping. I couldn't tell whether he had used it on Jay, or whether he had plans to introduce it to some part of my anatomy. I was not about to let him, and brought my baton up again for another strike, but he cowered away, half-running, half-leaping into a small set of bushes near the edge of the playground.

With great relief, I noticed another set of blue lights had joined ours. But I realised I couldn't hear anything. I couldn't hear the sirens on our car and I hadn't heard the other police car arrive. I glanced back. It was a carrier. The BSU serial we had heard on the radio earlier had come to our assistance.

Glancing back at Jay, I saw that the man who'd been kicking him had started to run, and now had two of the fully riot-clad BSU officers in hot pursuit.

The last guy, who had been pulling Jay from the car, had dropped his grip and was making to run off too. I didn't want to let him get away. I leapt forward and crashed into him. The top of my head smashed into his face as I carried out the least delicate rugby tackle ever attempted. My force caused the man to topple over onto the open car door. For a brief moment it seemed as if the door was going to give in at the hinges, but then it changed its mind and we were catapulted the other way. I ended up on my back, with the man I had dived at covering me like a blanket.

On the ground, trapped by 12 stone of athletic IC3 male, I tried to think of a way to use my baton, which I was still clinging on to. Before I made it that far, two men picked the assailant off of me and deposited him with great force, face first, onto the asphalt. I tilted my head backwards, and from my upside-down perspective, I saw that they were using zip-tie handcuffs to restrain him.

Looking back 'down', I saw Jay wrestle himself into an upright position, undo his seatbelt and climb out of the car. He must have been kicked in the head at least twice; a trickle of blood was running from his hair. He clutched his arm to his chest as he came over to me. He said something.

I still couldn't hear a thing.

He reached over to my radio, pressed the transmit button and said something, before cancelling the emergency mode.

Jay picked me up from the ground with his working arm. He opened the back door of the Mondeo, and dropped me in the back seat, leaving my legs still pointing out of the car. I sat up and felt instantly dizzy.

Gradually, as my adrenaline levels returned to normal, my hearing returned. Only then did I also realise that my colour vision had also been absent: I had been seeing the whole episode in a weird, super-slow-motion, sepia colour.

'You all right?' I could finally hear Jay ask.

'Yeah, I think so,' I said, leaning forward and placing my face in my hands. I found a piece of glass in my cheek, flicked it aside and returned my face to my hands. I had a dreadful headache.

'You're covered in blood. Ambulance on its way,' Jay summarised.

I twisted and leaned back into the back rest of the front seats. I was looking through the back window of the car. The whole area was swarming with police; at least half a dozen marked cars, a few rent-a-wrecks and two carriers had responded to my call for urgent assistance.

I couldn't hazard a guess at how long I had been sitting there like that, but after a while, I realised someone was talking to me. I had been zoning out, looking at the sea of blinking blue lights at the end of the short road.

'Say again?' I enquired.

Jay laughed.

He looked into my eyes, and I saw a flicker of . . . something I couldn't put my finger on.

'Thanks, Matt,' he said, before stepping aside, revealing a set of paramedics eager to take care of us.

Epilogue

Being a police officer is one of the most incredible jobs in the world.

It makes me laugh and cry and worry about the state of humanity. It encourages me to push myself beyond what I once thought was possible. It keeps me on my toes.

I've fought for my life. I've fought for the lives of others. I've saved lives, and I've felt people's heartbeats weaken and ebb away.

You can't do this job without investing something of yourself. For some officers, it's impossible to leave the role behind even when they've taken their uniforms off – but whatever happens, you have your colleagues around you, and my team members have become some of my best friends. Sometimes, in my more sentimental moments, I can't help but think of my colleagues as my band of brothers. A good thing, when your life occasionally depends on being able to trust them, and vice versa.

Policing can be stressful and emotionally draining, but it can also leave you buzzing. It can leave you feeling that you, personally, have contributed to making a tiny slice of London just a little bit better. Safer.

I remember the job I used to have. I remember sitting behind a computer screen all day, trying to sell people things they didn't want, in exchange for money they didn't have. A time when the measure of my success was a figure on a balance sheet at the end of each quarter. I'd take home a bonus (usually less than I, but more than my boss, felt I deserved), get pissed on ludicrously expensive wine and celebrate my 'successful' life. But all the while, I was miserable, because in the grand scheme of things, nothing I was doing really mattered.

Today's Me is embarrassed at the Me I used to be.

There are plenty of blogs on the Internet that are devoted to explaining how terrible it is to be a police officer, both in the Met and elsewhere. If you are one of those bloggers, I say: mate, if your current police job really is as bad as my pre-police job, *quit*. Get out of there. There are loads of people who are dreaming of donning a uniform and making a difference. If you hate it so much, make room for those who haven't yet burned out.

Being a police officer might not be the perfect job; given the hours we work and the mind-boggling amount of shite we have to deal with – well, let's just say you wouldn't become a police officer for the money. As in any large organisation, the bosses often '*don't get it*'. There's too much paperwork, too much health and safety, and too many new initiatives that spectacularly (and occasionally, hilariously) fail to reflect what it's actually like to be a police officer on the streets of London.

And yet, as I'm writing this, after coming home at the end of an absolute nasty-euphemism-for-female-genitalia of a shift, I'm sitting back with a cold beer, and thinking I wouldn't have it any other way.

Today, I made a difference.

I hope you liked my book.

Stay out of trouble.

Matt Delito PC592MD

Glossary and abbreviations

54 –   Form 54 is the form you fill in when a Met vehicle has to be taken
off the road for any reason: anything from a broken indicator
bulb to a blown engine. Hilariously, we are not allowed to do *any*
maintenance on the cars: we're not allowed to change a fuse or light-
bulb; we're not supposed to jump-start a car that has a flat battery;
they have even taken our jacks away so we can't change a flat tyre.
It's doubly ironic for the traffic coppers who have been trained to
take a car apart to look for stolen or illegal parts or modifications, so
clearly have all the mechanical skills needed to replace a little fuse. A
car is said to be '54'd' when it is waiting for a repair.

124D –   Form 124D is the domestic incident form; this is what is filled in
when we go to domestics. It's also used as radio slang for domestic
incidents – 'Delito, can you go to a one-two-four' generally means
that I'll be dodging kitchen knives the rest of the shift.

5090 –   A 5090 is a form, in triplicate, that is used when we do a stop and
search. Some officers are able to do these on electronic devices these
days, but most of us are still stuck with the forms. To 'do a 5090' is
to do a 'stop and search' or 'stop and account'.

ABH –   An 'assault occasioning Actual Bodily Harm', which means a serious
assault resulting in non-trivial injuries.

AED –   Automatic External Defibrillator: a machine that can be used to
reset the beating pattern of somebody's heart after a heart attack –
kind of like those paddles they use on TV (after they scream

'CLEAR', and you hear a zapping sound), except they're automatic, and a lot less dramatic.

AFO – Authorised Firearms Officer: the guys armed with loud weapons (guns) and sparkly weapons (tasers).

ATR – Automatic Time Recorder: an automatic stamping machine that is calibrated to only ever stamp the exact time it was used, along with a code for the police station that carried out the stamping.

Airwave – The system we use for our personal radios.

Angler – A burglar who uses a stick with a hook on it to steal things. Usually, anglers try to steal car keys that are left near the front door – they use their hook to grab the keys through the letterbox.

ATGATT – A motorcycling term meaning: All The Gear, All The Time. It refers to riders that choose to wear all their protective gear, even for very short rides, resisting the temptation to pop to the shops in their T-shirt and jeans.

Black Rat – Traffic police. So named because black rats eat their young, and traffic police will go after other police officers in traffic because they should know better. For a while, many police officers would place a small 'black rat' sticker in their rear windshield in the hope that other officers wouldn't pull them over. However, since that rumour took hold, lots of people started putting black rat stickers on their cars, and now you're as likely to get pulled over with such a sticker as not.

Body – Police slang for someone who is arrested. 'To get the body' means to be the arresting officer. 'We've got loads of bodies in this shift' means that lots of people have been conveyed to custody.

Brass – Anyone ranked Superintendent or above.

CARB – Collision and Accident Report Book: the little yellow booklet we fill in when we come across, er, collisions and accidents in traffic.

CHIMP – see PCSO

CPR – CardioPulmonary Resuscitation is an emergency procedure which is performed in an effort to manually preserve intact brain function until further measures are taken to restore spontaneous blood circulation and breathing in a person in cardiac arrest.

CPU – Case Progression Unit: officers who deal with cases currently in process.

CR –	Crime Reference number (see CRIS)
Crimint –	Criminal Intelligence is a database that keeps intelligence (intel) on all information we get from our informants. It's quite clever, and ranks the intel based on how reliable it is (ranging from 'known to be false' via 'from a usually reliable source' to 'known to be true because I saw it with my own eyes').
CRIS –	Crime Reporting Information System: the computer system onto which we log all criminal incidences. When you report a crime, you're given a Crime Reference number issued by our CRIS system.
CSI –	Crime Scene Investigator: usually called SOCOs in the Met. Some SOCOs will routinely refer to themselves as CSIs, because of the TV show, and because they believe it makes them sound cooler. To be fair, it kind of does.
Custodian –	The helmet-hat-thing that male Metropolitan Police officers are issued.
DPG –	Diplomatic Protection Group: the specialist officers, usually AFOs, tasked with protecting dignitaries, VIPs, heads of foreign states and other diplomats.
EAB –	Evidence and Action Book: a handy little 34-page booklet that has lots of aide-memoires in it, enabling overworked and slightly stressed police officers to do their jobs better.
Early Turn –	Working the early shift.
ELS –	Emergency Life Support. In the Met, officers aren't taught 'first aid' as such. If we come across anyone with an injury, we call an ambulance, and our job is simple: we do what we can to keep the victim alive until ambulance arrives.
F506 –	(only when written) Someone who is five foot six inches tall (see also M167).
Flat Cap –	The hat Met officers are issued for duties where wearing a Custodian is not appropriate.
FME –	**Forensic Medical Examiner.**
FPN(E) –	A traffic ticket where you, in addition to having to pay a fine, end up with a number of points on your licence.
FPN –	Fixed Penalty Notice – a traffic ticket.
GBH –	Grievous Bodily Harm: an assault where the attacker is intending to carry out serious or even life-changing injuries.

GFLB – Gravity Friction Lock Baton: the extendable batons police officers are issued.

Grade – Calls we attend are 'graded' based on how urgently we need to get to the location. Grade E or Echo is 'within 24 hours'. Grade S or Sierra is 'within the hour'. Graded I or India means 'however fast you can get there'. Our target within our borough is within 12 minutes of the call being logged in the system.

Graveyard Shift – The night shift.

GTP – Good To Police: areas where people are friendly to police. This also refers to shops that give a discount to uniformed officers.

Gun – In radio protocol a 'gun' is anything that can propel a bullet: rifles, cannons, handguns or homemade devices for propelling bullet-like things are all referred to as 'guns'.

Guv – Any officer with the Inspector rank or higher.

HEMS – Helicopter Emergency Medical Service: aka the London Air Ambulance charity. They have a helicopter and a load of rather fast ground-support vehicles, and only deal with trauma incidents: traffic, stabbings, shootings and falling accidents, mostly. If you have any spare money kicking about, give some to HEMS; the number of lives they save every year is absolutely astonishing.

Hendon – 'At Hendon' usually refers to the Peel Centre, also known as Hendon Police College. It is a huge training complex that serves as the main campus for the Metropolitan Police. It includes the advanced driving school, a load of classrooms and a series of gyms and training facilities. Interestingly, it is referred to as 'Hendon', even though Colindale tube station is much closer to the training centre itself.

IC – Identity Code: see *Identity codes* on page 291.

ICEFLO – One of the most ridiculous acronyms known to man. It stands for Immediate Capture of Evidence for Front Line Officers. It is much easier to just say 'Camera', which is what this means.

IRV – Incident Response Vehicle

Job – Police officers don't tend to refer to police as 'police'. Instead, we call it 'job'. If you're asking somebody else if they are also a police officer, you'd ask 'Are you job?' A police car is a 'job car'. A police dog is a 'job dog'. A police-issued mobile phone is a 'job phone'. You'll have spotted the pattern by now.

K9 unit – Dog unit: A *hilarious* pun on the word 'Canine', I'm sure. Shoot me now.

Knife – Much like anything that propels bullets is called 'gun', anything with a sharp edge or point is called a 'knife' when you're talking on the radio: this includes machetes, swords, injection needles, screwdrivers and corkscrews. If it cuts or stabs, it's a 'knife'.

LAS – London Ambulance Service

Late Turn – Working the late shift.

M167 – (only when written) someone who is one metre 67 centimetres tall (see also F506).

MDT – Mobile Data Terminal: A computer built into police cars. It contains (often inaccurate) maps, and is used by CAD operators to send tasks directly to our cars.

Met – The Metropolitan Police

MG-11 – The MG-11 form is used for general witness statements, whether taken from a victim, witness, informant or another police officer. It is always referred to as an 'MG-11', even though 'Em Gee Eleven' has one more syllable than 'Witness Statement', so you're not actually saving any time by using a form number rather than a description of what you're doing. If all of that makes perfect sense to you, you're ready to be a Metropolitan Police Constable. Congratulations.

MOP – A Member of the Public. Basically, anyone who is not a police officer.

Motorcycle Roadcraft – see Roadcraft

MPS – Metropolitan Police Service

Nick (noun) – usually 'The Nick': the police station.

Nick (verb) – to arrest somebody.

Non-Res – Non-residential: usually refers to commercial properties, such as in the context of 'non-residential burglary'.

Old Sweat – A police officer who has been in the job for a long time. Usually a term of endearment.

OST – Officer Safety Training: all training we get in being able to defend ourselves, perform arrests and assess various risks.

Panda – A police car, so called because they used to be black and white, which made them look a little bit like panda bears. The name stuck.

PB (also PPB) – see Pocketbook

PC – Police Constable: see also Ranks

PCSO – Extra uniformed people out there that can help be the police's eyes and ears, and take some tasks off our plate, but who ultimately don't have police powers (like powers of arrest etc). Sometimes referred to as CHIMPS, an acronym meaning Completely Helpless In Most Policing Situations. A bit cruel, perhaps, and I do think PCSOs are very useful, but ultimately, it's rather annoying when we have to go help out people who have 'Police' printed on their chest, without having the powers usually associated with the word.

PNC – The Police National Computer has a record of everybody who has been arrested in the past decade and a half, or so.

Pocketbook – (also PB, or PPB, for Police Pocketbook) The notebook you get issued when you join the police. This is where you write down any stops you do, keep a running log of your shifts, and do a lot of arse-covering in case you have to use any force that isn't covered in any other pieces of paperwork. Personally, I like to keep a quick note of all the reference numbers from other forms here, too: the serial numbers on tickets I issue, the numberplates of cars I check, and the details of people I've spoken to. Whenever you end up in court, you rely heavily on your pocketbook. If it's not written down, it didn't happen. When you finish your pocketbook, it gets filed away for ten years. Lose your pocketbook, and you could face rather serious disciplinary action.

PR – Personal Radio

PTT – The Push To Talk button does what it says on the tin: push the button to transmit, and release it again to end your transmission.

Q Car – An unmarked police car. Usually, these vehicles have concealed radio antennae, hidden lights and tucked-away sirens. These days, some of the Q cars are so well camouflaged that even if you were to inspect one that was parked, you might not be able to identify it as a police car. The name Q car derives from the Second World War expression 'Q Ship'. These were heavily armed merchant ships with concealed weaponry, designed to lure submarines into making surface attacks. This gave Q ships the chance to open fire and sink them.

QT – Saying the Q-word meaning 'the opposite of loud' is bad luck in this job; whenever someone exclaims 'Boy, is it quiet today', it invariably means that the rest of the shift descends into a shitstorm of historical proportions. The last time someone mentioned the Q-word over the radio, the riots broke out a few hours later. QT stands for Quiet Time.

Rank – When you start working as a police officer, you usually enter as a police constable – you can then work your way up the ranks. For an overview of the positions, see *Police Ranks* on page 292.

Refs – Refreshment: When taking a tea or food break, you're said to be 'on refs'.

Res – Residential: places where people live; the opposite of Non-Res.

Roadcraft – The name of the advanced driving book we use as our textbook in the police. You can buy it from bookstores, if you're curious.

RPG – Rocket Propelled Grenade, if you're an avid gamer. In the context of the Met, however, it's the Royal Protection Group: the specialist officers, usually AFOs as well, who are tasked with protecting members of the Royal Family.

RTC – Road Traffic Collision

Sarge – see Sergeant

SC – see Special Constable

Sergeant – The rank above Constable

Skipper – see Sergeant

SMT – Senior Management Team

SOCO – Scene of Crimes Officer; like CSI, but more British.

Special Constable – Police constables who volunteer their time to work alongside regular officers. They usually have a 'real' job in addition to being volunteer officers. They use the same equipment and have the same police powers as myself.

Stick – see also Gun and Knife: a stick is anything that can be used to hit someone with: a piece of plank, a baseball bat or, yes, a stick.

Sticking – Hitting someone with a baton or truncheon.

Tit – see Custodian

TLA – Three Letter Acronym

Top hat – see Custodian

Tour of Duty – A shift at work.

Trojan – Armed police, see also *AFO*.

Tug – To pull over a car.

TWOC – Take Without Owner's Consent in instances of car theft.

VIWS – Victims, Informants, Witnesses and Suspects.

White Notes – The training paperwork you get when you learn everything you need to know to be a police officer. Why they are called 'white notes', I have never been able to figure out.

Identity codes

IC stands for Identity Code. They are used to describe the apparent ethnic background of Victims, Informants, Witnesses and Suspects (collectively known as VIWS). If it isn't immediately clear what IC code your VIWS are, you take your best guess.

IC1 – White person, northern European
IC2 – White person, Mediterranean/Hispanic
IC3 – African/Afro-Caribbean person
IC4 – Indian, Pakistani, Nepalese, Maldivian, Sri Lankan, Bangladeshi or any other (South) Asian person
IC5 – Chinese, Japanese or South-East Asian person
IC6 – Arab person

Police ranks

1. Police Constable (PC)
2. Police Sergeant (PS)
3. Inspector (Insp)
4. Chief Inspector (C/Insp)
5. Superintendent (Supt/Super)
6. Chief Superintendent (C/Supt)
7. Commander (Cdr)
8. Deputy Assistant Commissioner (DAC)
9. Assistant Commissioner (AC)
10. Deputy Commissioner (D/Comm)
11. Commissioner (Comm)

Acknowledgements

This book could not have happened without the incredible support I've received throughout the process of it coming about – the support from Kat Hannaford at Gizmodo, and Rachel Faulkner and Scott Pack at The Friday Project has been absolutely magnificent. Thank you so much. A big thanks also to Katie May, for making me look all manner of wholesome on the cover of this book. I wish I were that good looking!

Confessions of a Police Constable is part of the bestselling 'Confessions' series. Also available:

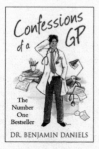

Confessions of a GP
by Dr. Benjamin Daniels

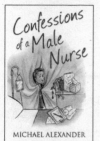

Confessions of a Male Nurse
by Michael Alexander

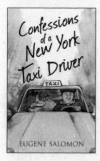

Confessions of a New York Taxi Driver
by Eugene Salomon

Look out for *Confessions of a Showbiz Reporter* and *Confessions of an Undercover Cop*, coming soon.